Smart Health

Smart Health

WHAT TODAY'S DOCTORS AREN'T TELLING YOU

The Series

Dr. Craig C. Koehler

Kindle Edition

Disclaimer: The information provided in the eBook or physical copy of this book, including on the website www.koehlerwellness.com, is intended for your general knowledge only and is not a substitute for professional medical advice or treatment for specific medical conditions. Always seek the advice of your general practitioner, physician, or other qualified health-care provider with any questions you may have regarding a medical condition or when starting any health- or nutritional-related treatment. This information is not intended to diagnose, treat, cure, or prevent any disease. Never disregard medical advice or delay in seeking treatment because of something you have read in this book or on our website. Any products recommended have been thoroughly researched; however, as with all products sold, you are always recommended to do your own research, including consulting with a qualified medical or health-care provider.

ISBN: 0998091804
ISBN-13: 9780998091808

Smart Health Publishing
Huntington Beach, CA

Formatted by Debbie Lum
debbie@debbiestevenlum.com

www.KoehlerWellness.com

For exclusive updates, visit:
www.SmartHealthExperience.com

Dedication

To my loving parents, Augie and Rita.
You have given me such love and support beginning at the start of my formative years that still continues into my adult years. I appreciate you, and I love you.

Contents

Foreword

My life has been a long road of self-discovery. Growing up a sickly child in the health-care system as we all know it today led me directly to the path I am on now. As much as I wished I could have been a famous rock-and-roll star or even a bad-boy biker, I chose to become a chiropractor. Had I not chosen this path, I am quite certain I would be a very unhealthy adult by now. This path has led me to a deep understanding of health, healing, and the dangers of the American health-care "system" as we know it today.

The fact that medical mistakes and errors in our current health-care system are now the third leading cause of death in the United States is unbelievable to me. **We are currently listed at number thirty-three of the healthiest countries in the world—that's right, thirty-three!** I must admit, as an American, that is quite embarrassing.

Big Pharma has got a death grip on our nation, and it isn't going to let go anytime soon. You must get educated and you must get informed about your health; it could literally make the difference between life or death in our health-care system.

This book is designed to inform and educate you in ways that can lead you on a path to improving your health and overall well-being. I believe each chapter will give you a better understanding of what the problems are today and the solutions you will need to overcome them.

I realize it is no easy task to turn your health around. I realize that you have not ever been taught in detail how to be healthy and what to actually do to stay healthy. Even worse, we may have already become addicted to the poisons that some call food, or which are better described as junk food.

I have worked one-on-one with my patients for over twenty-five years. I look at my patients as if they are children of my office. I am here to protect them, look after them, and many times, learn from them and their journeys as well. I have seen families grow and send their children and even their grandchildren for me to care for.

I have dedicated my life and my career to helping my patients; you are my world.

My Personal Story

When I was twelve years old, I would ride my bike home from school every day. I loved that bike! It was one of those ten-speed bikes, you know, with the racing handlebars. One sunny afternoon, I was almost home—just four blocks to go—and I must have hit that one big bump in the sidewalk where the tree root raises the sidewalk up. I lost my balance, fell off my bike, and I hit my head right on the cement. I was knocked out cold. Fortunately, Mr. Hamilton, our neighborhood mailman, saw the whole thing. He was a big burly guy; he rushed over, scooped me up, laid me down in the back of his mailman truck, and took me straight home to my parents. My parents were obviously very concerned and immediately took me to the emergency room; thankfully, I seemed to check out OK.

It was about a year later, though, that I became that kid in school who was always coughing, sneezing, and blowing his nose. As a result, I had a hard time fitting in with the other kids, especially the girls. It seems the kids weren't all that interested in a boy who was sneezing and blowing his nose all the time. I remember hearing the word *icky* being used on a regular basis. Literally every day I would have to bring my "hanky" with me to school. I was constantly sneezing and constantly blowing my nose. I knew something was wrong—I knew the other kids didn't have to blow their noses and constantly use a hanky—but I didn't understand why, and it would be years before I would understand the connection.

As time went on, our family doctor began prescribing more and more medications. Initially it was the antihistamines; they seemed to work for a while, but I needed more and more of them. Soon I was popping antihistamines like they were M&Ms. Not to mention they made me very drowsy. Next, it was the antibiotics, because it was now "obvious" I must have an infection...every month. Of course, that didn't help.

Next, I was prescribed allergy shots. I would ride my bicycle to the allergy doctor's office twice a week and get shots in both arms for two years! I remember absolutely hating those shots. You guessed it: that didn't help either.

So, years later, I was still the kid in school who was sneezing and blowing his nose all day long. Eventually, our doctor decided that my tonsils were now infected, and they needed to be removed from my body. Do you know that your tonsils are part of your immune system? Well, it's true. If you can help it, don't let anybody cut out and remove any part of your immune system. Keep your tonsils!

What I Had Learned by Age Seventeen

By the time I was seventeen years old, I had already learned a lot about health. Here's what I knew to be true: that constantly taking medications, injecting needles into your arms, and especially undergoing surgery were *not* the answers to a healthy body. **This began my lifelong journey of studying health.**

I remember one early morning before school, it was really cold out, and I was taking the trash cans out to the front of the house. I'm so thankful my parents had me do chores. I lifted this one really heavy trash can that was probably too full, and I remember immediately feeling pain in my lower back. The next morning my back pain was worse, much worse. I remember complaining to my mom about my lower back pain, and thank God, she took me to their chiropractor. My father was in construction, and my parents would go to the chiropractor from time to time. The very next day, I was in the chiropractor's office, and I saw this nerve chart on the wall that shows how the brain sends all of its messages and signals from the brain to the brain stem and then down into the spinal cord. From the spinal cord the nerves branch out, kind of like how a tree branch will branch out from the trunk of a tree. These nerves connect and communicate to every part of the body, including the lower back, legs, neck, arms, and your body's internal organs as well. So, I asked about the sinuses. I distinctly remember our chiropractor, Dr. Rita Schroeder, showing me that there was an actual nerve connection from my neck going directly to the sinuses. I swear to you, right then and there, **it was as if a light bulb had been turned on!**

Now, I had been committed to becoming an engineer, or more than likely, an architect. I was really impressed by the architect Frank Lloyd Wright. I had been drawing plans and doing basic home design for years, and I really loved it. But when that light bulb went on inside my head, I knew that I had to study more about health and how this nervous system controls our body. I was so fascinated at how all these nerves worked, and I wondered if that fall when I hit my head on the cement at age twelve could be **the real reason** why I had been having all these allergy and sinus problems for so many years. So I went to college, and by the time I was twenty-six, I was a licensed doctor of chiropractic!

Now, the Work Begins

What I've learned about health, nutrition, exercise, and especially making positive changes to your life and your lifestyle, has truly been amazing. I've learned that you really **can turn your health around** and become healthy again. By applying basic principles of health and more advanced high-tech principles we have discovered today, you can easily lose weight, build muscle, and get off some—hopefully all—of the medications that many times aren't necessary. To date, I have not been on an antihistamine or an antibiotic medication in well over twenty years.

It has been a long journey, and not without my own personal struggles and challenges. Before I turned forty years old, I hired a personal trainer. I figured when I turned forty I wanted to be in tip-top shape. I did my research and I found a guy who worked with me two to three times a week. When I turned forty, I was in awesome shape, thanks to Jason! He was cool guy, a rocker, and we got along quite well. The real reasons I hired him were: 1) He was not a young guy in his early twenties. No offense to the young kids in their twenties, but I like taking my advice from someone that has a few more miles on his odometer. 2) He was ripped. I mean, he was shredded—the guy was muscular, yes—but what he really had was the abs! To me, having abs is what takes the most discipline. Not just with your exercise and workouts, but more importantly, with your nutrition. That was the guy I wanted to learn from. We must have worked together for at least a year or so, and then I decided that I was all set and disciplined with my workouts and my nutrition routine, so we parted ways. In hindsight, that wasn't my brightest decision. I continued to work out here and there, but not with the same intensity or the same frequency. Slowly, and sadly, I stopped working out. My nutrition slowly worsened, too. I mean, it wasn't bad, but it certainly wasn't good either. I share my personal struggle with sugar addiction in a later chapter.

Then, when I was getting close to fifty, I thought to myself, "Hey, I should get back to work on this body of mine, and I can do it again! That way when I turn fifty, I will be in excellent shape again." So, I made an agreement with myself to start working out and to clean up my nutrition. But this time I was going to do it all on my own. Well, I'm not too sure what happened, but I somehow woke up just after turning fifty-three, and I hadn't done a damn thing. I hadn't even started. I joined and then later started a support group that made a world of difference! Be sure to read the chapter "**Your Support Team**."

I Had Been Telling My Patients, but What About Me?

Heck, none of my clothes were fitting anymore. My pants were getting super tight in the waist, and I would have to keep the top button unbuttoned to wear them with my belt covering it so I wouldn't have to buy new dress slacks. I don't think anyone ever noticed, but I knew. I was having a problem with my weight. My body just wasn't as young as it used to be, and frankly, I was tired from working all day long in the office!

I knew I was getting flabby and my muscle tone was slowly going away. When you finally get to that point, that's when you know you have to do something about it. That is the time when you are finally going to commit to this next journey in your life. So, I did some research, and what I found was that if I used an actual "system"- something where I didn't have to think too much about it, something that I could stick to, something simple—then maybe, just maybe, I could get this body turned around and get back in shape. As I'm writing this today, I have stayed very committed and continue to be "all in." Almost three years down the road, my physique is in pretty darn good shape. Let's just say that I'm never shy about taking my shirt off anymore. Be sure to read the chapter on "**Mobility and Increasing Your Energy**."

When Your Family Members Die

What hit me the hardest, though, was the untimely deaths of some family members. One of my cousins died of pancreatic cancer. Do you know that the statistics on pancreatic cancer are that only 5 percent of people with this diagnosis will live five years? So that means 100 percent will die. Even the richest of the rich, Steve Jobs, couldn't buy his way to health with pancreatic cancer. Now, I don't know all of the details of my cousin's or Steve Jobs' diagnoses or the contributing factors to their diseases, but what I can tell you is that there is a direct link between a high level of sugar intake and pancreas problems that include diabetes and cancer, too. Be sure to check out the chapter on **"Sugar and Junk Food, the Real Gateway Drugs."**

Another family member certainly had an eating disorder and was very overweight. I don't know the exact numbers, but I'm sure it was in the 300+ range. Bless her heart, with very good intentions she knew this was affecting her health, and she became committed to doing the right thing and losing weight. With much research, she decided that gastric bypass surgery would certainly be the answer to her prayers. Initially, the surgery went well—or so they thought. She was not able to eat anything or keep anything down, and that included water. Perhaps the surgeon didn't leave enough room for anything to get into and stay in the stomach. She vomited everything back up. After consulting with the surgeon on numerous occasions, she was assured this was not uncommon; she was sent home and told not to worry. Weeks passed, and she was still unable to keep anything down. Due to an electrolyte imbalance from dehydration, she had a heart attack and slipped into a coma. She never came out of the coma, and about a year later she passed away, dying at the very young age of thirty-four, directly due to complications from the gastric bypass surgery. I highly recommend reading the chapter on "**Water: Your Core Energy Source"** so you can begin to understand the importance of water in your life. As you might imagine, this devastated the entire family to include losing the house they called home.

These two very personal stories are from my own family members, not something that I read about in the newspaper or saw on the evening news on TV. I actually *know* these people. Well, I knew them.

Why I Wrote This Book

I know what it is like to not have your health. I lived that life. I know that had I not chosen this path, there is no way I would have the abundance of health that I do today. As I am still in private practice working with patients one-on-one,

I see the personal struggles that my patients have with their own health. I see exactly how our health-care "system" operates. I see how the HMO insurance plans typically treat their insured. I see how the Medicare and the Obamacare patients are treated in our health-care system. I have learned so much from my patients over the last twenty-five years that I know that what I am teaching you in this book is exactly **what today's doctors aren't telling you**.

So, let me tell you about my vision. My vision is to create a community of health-minded and healthy people. People that are committed to their health. People that have come to realize that our health-care "system," and our health in the United States is not what it could and should be. People that understand that we were never taught how to be healthy or given the tools to be healthy. We were never taught this when we were kids, and we certainly aren't being taught this as adults. Even though today we have complete access to all of this information, and it is literally at our fingertips thanks to our computers, we are still getting sicker and sicker, fatter and fatter, and taking more and more medications. Just look around you: our friends, our family members, and our community are all on prescription medications; there are drugstores on every corner. People are overweight, stressed out, and filling their mouths with junk food. Cancer, heart disease, diabetes, obesity, and metabolic diseases are running rampant in our society, and are slowly killing us each and every day. Be sure to read the chapter "**The Common Diseases, Big Pharma—Kill or Cure?**"

It has and always will be my mission to educate, motivate, and inspire people to improve their health, even if it is only one little step at a time. You see, I want to surround myself with people who are healthy and who have come to realize that no one is coming to save them or their health. You must be involved in your health; it is one of the biggest commodities you will ever have. You are ultimately in charge and in control of your own health. I want to help people who really want to be healthy to be on top of their games, getting off the unnecessary medications, eating correctly, getting rid of excess weight, and exercising. I want to create a world of "**health warriors.**"

So, take a moment, go to our website at www.koehlerwellness.com, and let us know about your health and what you are struggling with, and we will find a way to help you! You have my word on it. You can contact our office at 714.846.3544 or e-mail at info@koehlerwellness.com.

PART I

The Problems We Face and Your Health

Pain Killers Are Killing You

Americans consume 80 percent of the world's pain pills in the form of legal prescription pain medications. Painkiller medication overdoses have caused more deaths than traffic accidents every year since the year 2000. Almost half of Americans—44 percent of them—know someone personally who has been addicted to prescription painkillers. **Have I got your attention?**

The International Association for the Study of Pain's definition states: "Pain is an unpleasant sensory and emotional experience associated with actual or potential tissue damage." **In medical diagnosis, pain is merely a symptom.**

However, in dealing with an injury or pain, you must always pay attention and search for the **cause** of the pain. When treating pain with medications or cortisone shots, you are simply masking the root cause of the pain and treating the pain only. What this does is prolong the appropriate treatment, and the cause of the pain continues and usually gets worse. I explain to patients that typically the longer ago the injury originally occurred, the longer it will take to stabilize and/or correct what is actually **causing the pain**. The truth of the matter is that many for injuries that we sustain in our lives, we are simply not able to overcome and correct to 100 percent preinjury status.

This reminds me of a patient long ago who was an actual repo man. He would work throughout the night picking up vehicles from people who would not make their payments. He loved his work! The excitement, the intrigue, and apparently, the pay was pretty good, too. One night out repossessing a car, he actually took a bullet in the back. He literally got shot in the back! Had he not had on a bulletproof vest, he would have probably died. Not only did he lose interest in being a repo man after that, but his back will never be the same as a result, and he continues with chronic pain.

Take professional athletes who have developed a very high level of physical skill. Normally when they sustain an injury, they will almost immediately begin a rehab program working on the actual cause of their pain to resolve their injury as quickly as possible. Although, I'm sure there are countless stories of professional athletes who are doped-up on medications and who play injured so that they can play in the big game. I also recognize the consequences of addiction to pain-killing drugs and medications. The history books are full of top-notch athletes who have had their careers cut short due to injuries and pain-killing medication addictions. Bottom line: the stronger your body is, and the faster you begin working on the cause of that injury, the better off you will be. The San Francisco 49ers' Jerry Rice is a prime example of keeping his body strong throughout his lengthy carrier.

Pain Is Natural to Our Bodies

Pain is a natural part of body functions. It motivates us from dangerous and damaging situations and protects a damaged body part while it heals. It also helps to protect us from similar experiences in the future. Most pain resolves once the noxious stimulus is removed and the body has healed. Sometimes, though, pain arises in the absence of any detectable stimulus, damage, or disease. Simple pain medications can be useful in most of these cases. However, these pain medications simply mask the cause of the problem, which can actually interfere with healing and many times leads to stronger and stronger pain medications.

Pain is the most common reason for physician consultation in most developed countries. Pain is a major symptom in many medical conditions and can interfere with a person's quality of life and general functioning. Psychological factors such as social support, hypnotic suggestion, excitement, or distraction can significantly affect pain's intensity or unpleasantness.

In my private practice, we primarily treat musculoskeletal conditions, and those are almost always associated with pain. I know that when pain gets bad, it can literally stop a person in his or her tracks, whether it be headaches, neck pain, back pain, sciatica pain, shoulder pain, or knee pain. I've had women tell me that their sciatic pain is worse than childbirth, and I have literally seen grown men cry due to their crippling lower-back pain. I've had patients tell me their headaches are so bad they wished they could cut their heads off. I personally have had a few accidents myself over the years and have periodically felt some significant pain; it really is no picnic.

Frequently, an old injury will flare up while you are doing yard work, housework, even just bending or lifting at the wrong time. This pain will slow your life down and lead to frustration, depression, and almost always irritability too.

Pain and Painkillers Are Big Business

Pain and pain medication in the United States are big, big business! In the medical and pharmacology industries, they have invented a new doctor category that is specifically and primarily just for treating pain. The "pain management" specialist essentially prescribes higher doses and stronger pain medications for your pain, whatever that may be. The problem with this new trend is that treating your injuries with pain medication is not getting to the cause of the problem and leads to:

1. Postponing appropriate treatment to actually heal the injury.
2. Easily becoming addicted to pain medications.
3. Building up a tolerance to the pain medications, needing more and more to combat the pain.
4. Developing some of the serious side effects from taking pain medications.
5. Eventually being cut off from the medication and referred to drug rehabilitation by the pain management doctor once it is determined that you are now addicted to pain medication.

The problem all along is that the cause of your condition has never been determined and treated appropriately. I have seen this exact scenario literally thousands of times in private practice.

I don't necessarily blame the patients, as they are simply believing in and following their doctors' recommendations. You must, however, understand the system. Typically, the doctor will do the very easiest, simplest—and in my opinion—laziest form of treatment, and that is the prescription pad. Patients must learn to be their own best "patient advocate," and do some research and ask questions. This video, "Drug Companies Putting Profits

Above Patients," will help you understand the motives behind Big Pharma and their doctors. Here is the video link: http://bit.ly/2CgDt9oGreed.

The Most Commonly Reported Pain Conditions

According to the National Institute of Health, the statistics reveal that low-back pain was the most common pain complaint at (28 percent), followed by knee pain (19 percent), severe headache or migraine pain (16 percent), neck pain (15 percent), shoulder pain (9 percent), finger pain (7 percent), and hip pain (7 percent).

Back pain is the leading cause of disability in Americans under forty-five years old. More than twenty-six million Americans between the ages of twenty and sixty-four experience frequent back pain: http://wb.md/1pyJ39W.

Adults with low back pain are typically in worse overall physical and mental health than people who do not have low-back pain. They will report they are three times as likely to be in fair or poor health, and more than four times as likely to experience serious psychological distress, versus people without low-back pain.

Chronic Pain

Chronic pain is pain that lasts much longer than would be expected from the original problem or injury. When pain becomes chronic, your body may react in several ways. Chronic pain may be characterized by abnormal brain hormones, low energy, mood disorder, muscle pain, and impaired mental and physical performance. Chronic pain worsens as neurochemical changes increase your sensitivity to pain. Frequently you begin to have pain in other parts of your body that do not normally hurt. Before long, everything hurts.

Living with chronic or long-term pain is a tremendous burden. But when you have chronic pain and depression, the burden gets even heavier.

Chronic pain can lead to depression, and depression magnifies pain. It makes it difficult to cope with everyday life and living. Chronic pain can also prevent sleep and cause you to wake up frequently at night. Lack of sleep results in daytime fatigue and, of course, low productivity. The ongoing pain will lead to irritability and stress in your relationships and feelings of being overwhelmed.

What Happens with Chronic Pain and Depression?

If you have chronic pain and depression, you have plenty of company. Depression is one of the most common psychological issues facing people who suffer from chronic pain, and it often complicates the patient's condition and treatment. Consider these statistics:

- According to the American Pain Foundation, about thirty-two million people in the United States report they have pain lasting longer than one year.
- About half of the population who complain of chronic pain to their doctors are also depressed.
- On average, 65 percent of depressed people also complain of pain.
- People whose pain limits their independence are especially likely to get depressed.

Americans Consume 80 Percent of the World's Pain Pills as Prescription Drugs

Americans consume 80 percent of the world's supply of painkillers. More than 110 tons of pure, addictive opiates are consumed every year as this country's prescription-drug-abuse epidemic explodes. It has been estimated that approximately 4.7 million people are addicted to prescription painkillers, representing a 300 percent increase since 1999. Here is a link that helps to explain it: http://dailym.ai/1Gt7WyG. This video link from ABC will also help you understand this epidemic: http://abcn.ws/1U3H6kN

Here are some cold hard facts from the Center for Disease Control (CDC) and Business Insider:

- In 2015, drug overdoses took more lives every year (since 2009) than traffic accidents.
- In 2010, more people age twelve and older abused or were dependent on prescription painkillers than cocaine, heroin, stimulants, and sedatives combined.
- Deaths from prescription painkillers (opioid), in the United States have more than tripled since the year 2000 and so have the sales of these drugs.

- In 2009, there were 500,000 emergency room visits due to people abusing prescription painkillers.
- In 2010, one in every twenty people in the United States age twelve and older reported using prescription painkillers nonmedically—that's twelve million people—and half of all deaths from painkillers also involve another drug, like alcohol or another pharmaceutical pill.
- The annual cost to health insures due to nonmedical use of prescription painkillers is $72.5 billion.
- In 2011, the Centers for Disease Control and Prevention reported that the rate of antidepressant use in the United States rose by 400 percent between 1988 and 2008.
- During 2014, a total of 47,055 drug overdose deaths occurred in the United States.
- From 1999 to 2013, the number of painkillers prescribed and sold in the United States has nearly quadrupled, and overdose of deaths have quadrupled.

It is easy to see this is a very serious problem. These findings indicate that the opioid- and painkiller-overdose epidemics are worsening. There is a need for continued action to prevent this abuse, dependence, and resulting death by overdose. The numbers say it all. Distribution of morphine—the primary ingredient in the most popular of painkillers—has exploded 600 percent from 1997 to 2007, according to the US Drug Enforcement Agency. The Centers for Disease Control and Prevention have called accidental overdoses of prescription medication "an epidemic," thanks to the doctors who are more and more willing to hand out prescriptions to these drugs, the pharmacists who are filling the prescriptions, and the patients who are "suffering." In 2015, the CDC data reveals the bottom line; prescribed and legal pain-killing medications are now killing more people than cocaine and heroin *combined*! **These are "legal medications."**

Now Referred to As Generation Rx

Research in the *Journal of Public Policy & Marketing* attributes much of the pharmaceutical abuse problem to the perception that all prescription drugs are safe because they were prescribed by a doctor. With a prescription medication, you are exempt from the stigma that is attached to illegal drugs. Prescription drugs are seen as blessed by a doctor and a trusted institution, the FDA. Increasingly aggressive advertising by drug companies directly to consumers floods parents and children with messages that these substances are safe, popular, and beneficial. Here is a link to learn more: http://bit.ly/2o4fm8yAdvertisingDrugs.

This positive perception of pharmaceuticals is heightened by drug companies' advertisements in television and media ads that has led to a culture of a "pill-for-every-ill" approach to health care in the United States and has some officials calling for an end to consumer drug advertising. We must pay attention to our youth with high levels of anxiety and not underestimate the risks of prescription drugs and the likelihood of abuse in all ages.

In the meantime, of course, the epidemic continues to grow like wildfire! This year, the CDC statistics state that in 2014 the five states with the highest rates of drug overdose were: West Virginia (35.5 deaths per 100,000), New Mexico (27.3), New Hampshire (26.2), Kentucky (24.7), Ohio (24.6), Nevada (22.4), and Utah (21.9).

States with significant increases in the rate of drug overdose deaths from 2013 to 2014 include Alabama, Georgia, Illinois, Indiana, Maine, Maryland, Massachusetts, Michigan, New Hampshire, New Mexico, North Dakota, Ohio, Pennsylvania, and Virginia. http://1.usa.gov/1PScwrW.

Unfortunately, accidental overdose usually only makes national headlines if a celebrity overdoses, not our close friends, our neighbors, or our own family members.

The most common occurrences, however, involve normal Americans who turn to the medicine chest for relief of pain that probably started from an injury either recent or from the past. We may start with an over-the-counter medication and eventually turn to prescription medications, instead of actually working on the root cause of the condition. Let's face it, it is so much easier to simply pop some pills to make everything feel better, right? Typically, when you present to your family physician complaining of pain, you will leave with a prescription for pain medication. It really is just that simple, and this has become expected.

In my opinion, instead of the prescription pad immediately being pulled out, there should be time spent on investigating the actual *cause* of the pain instead of simply masking it with pain medications. Am I completely crazy, or does this make any sense?

As more people get their hands on these dangerous and addicting drugs, more are taking them to get high. Their drug abuse leads to alarming increases in deaths each year that have now outnumbered heroin and cocaine combined. This epidemic is ruining the lives and families of Americans and profiting the medical system.

Prescription Drugs, Doctor Prescribed and Pharmacy Filled

"We've become a society of wusses," says Long Island, New York, pharmacist Dr. Howard Levin. "Doctors are too willing to hand out prescription painkillers and Americans have the highest incidence of use of hydrocodone and oxycodone in the world," Dr. Levin states in an interview by the BBC News. Personally, I love this guy because he is willing to stand up and tell it like it is!

Death due to drug overdose can also be the result of mixing prescribed medications with other drugs, whether they are prescription or illegal, and that includes alcohol and over interactions. Please use the following link as a reference for checking potential drug interactions: http://bit.ly/2El74nLDrugInteractions. If this link were to even save even one person's life, I would consider my work here a complete success.

The main side effect of these medications is that they depress the central nervous system. Opioid-based painkillers, sedatives, hypnotics, and alcohol depress, slow down, and can eventually stop our breathing. With an unintentional overdose or when these are mixed together, they slow down the breathing until you simply stop breathing altogether. Personally, I am a big fan of breathing.

Mixing illicit, prescription, or over-the-counter medications can be very dangerous, and patients should always rule out drug interactions with either their health-care provider, a pharmacist, or do not forget about our friend, Google. The use of prescription medications with illegal drugs or alcohol can produce an unpredictable and fatal response.

The following outlines the deaths of notable celebrities and athletes who have had prescription medications, drugs, or alcohol implicated in their deaths:

- Prince: fentanyl (opioid overdose)
- Michael Jackson: propofol, midazolam, lidocaine, Valium, lorazepam

- Whitney Houston: cocaine, Flexeril, Xanax, Benadryl, marijuana
- Heath Ledger: oxycodone, hydrocodone, alprazolam, Valium, Temazepam, Doxylamine
- Joan Rivers: propofol
- Jeff Hanneman: liver cirrhosis due to alcohol
- Amy Winehouse: alcohol poisoning
- Erica Blasberg, professional golfer: hydrocodone, tramadol, alprazolam, codeine
- Billy Mays: cocaine use with heart disease
- Philip Seymour Hoffman: heroin, cocaine, benzodiazepines, and amphetamine
- Anna Nicole Smith: chloral hydrate, benzodiazepines
- Chris Farley: morphine, cocaine, fluoxetine
- Margeaux Hemingway: phenobarbital
- Kurt Cobain: lethal dose of heroin (suicide)
- River Phoenix: heroin and cocaine overdose
- Richard Burton: complications due to alcoholism
- Truman Capote: alcohol and multiple drug intoxication
- John Belushi: heroin and cocaine overdose
- Elvis Presley: cardiac arrhythmia caused from overdose of codeine, Valium, morphine, and Demerol
- Howard Hughes: kidney failure due to complication of chronic use of aspirin; physician administered an overdose of codeine, leading to liver failure.
- Bruce Lee: meprobamate, Equagesic (painkiller) aspirin
- Jimi Hendrix: alcohol and barbiturate overdose
- Jim Morrison: multiple drugs and alcohol abuse, heroin overdose
- Janis Joplin: heroin and alcohol overdose
- Judy Garland: barbiturate overdose
- Lenny Bruce: morphine
- Marilyn Monroe: barbiturate overdose
- Billie Holiday: alcohol and heroin abuse
- Tommy Dorsey: sedative overdose
- Brittany Murphy: multiple drug intoxication
- Coco Chanel: heroin and opiate abuse leading to heart complications
- Bobby Hatfield: cocaine-induced heart attack

- Christina Onassis: Dexedrine (diet pills), barbiturates leading to pulmonary edema
- Lenny Bruce: heroin overdose (reportedly)

Medical Conditions Do Require Pain Relief

There are many chronic medical conditions that absolutely do require continual pain relief. With this continued demand and the awareness of pain medication and resulting addiction, we have developed and formulated a topical pain relief cream. This product, Pain Relief *Now*, has been developed under the strictest of guidelines, clinically tested, and is now being introduced to consumers. It is an exceptional product, a topical pain relief cream that is nothing short of amazing!

The list of ingredients has been well researched and are fast acting, soothing, healing, and anti-inflammatory; it is very simple to use. You open the jar and rub the cream right on the area of pain. You should feel some relief almost immediately. We do recommend repeating the use three to four times per day or as needed.

Pain Relief *Now* is available on our website, www.koehlerwellness.com/pain-relief-now/, and on Amazon: http://bit.ly/2El1Uo1PainReliefNow

In the next chapter on common diseases I will discuss Big Pharma - "Kill or Cure?" which was a phrase my grandfather used as he described to me what it was like taking my grandmother in for her cancer treatment.

The Common Diseases, Big Pharma—Kill or Cure?

After five years of reviewing seven thousand medical studies, a team of top scientists from around the world have concluded that your nutrition and your weight directly affect whether or not you will get cancer. The researchers cite "convincing" evidence that excess body fat can cause many different types of common cancers, including those affecting the breast, bowel, and pancreas. The research also links consumption of alcohol, red meat, and processed meat to an increased risk of cancer. "It should come as no real surprise that excess body fat is associated with cancer, since many dietary (nutritional) factors that protect against cancer are probably absent in the diet of an overweight or obese person," said Daniel Hoffman, professor of nutritional sciences at Rutgers University in Newark, New Jersey.

Cancer, Heart Disease, Diabetes, and Obesity

If you start connecting the dots, it will become quite apparent that your lifestyle gets directly connected to not only the Big Four diseases, which are cancer, heart disease, diabetes, and obesity, but most of the chronic health and metabolic diseases as well.

Your lifestyle. Is it possible that we can literally be our own worst enemies regarding our own health and the health of our families? You want to and need to adopt an active lifestyle that is centered with good clean nutrition, plenty of exercise, getting enough sleep, hydrating your body with clean water, staying away from sugar and junk food, and looking to the cause of any physical pains.

If you follow this pattern of living, your body will be healthier, your self-image will improve, you will look better, and you will feel better too. This type of lifestyle leads to living a life of abundance and richness in all aspects. Isn't this the life we all want to live?

When you choose—and it is a choice—*not* to live this type of lifestyle, your body slowly gets sicker and sicker. It becomes more vulnerable to infection and injury, and as a result, you end up gaining weight and eventually taking medications. When you combine unhealthy eating, lifestyle stress, and alcohol, the results lead to difficulty sleeping. Now you have created a cocktail for disease. We are going to take a look at the most popular diseases and medications, and how much Americans are spending on them each year because of our poor lifestyle choices

Cancer

What a horrible word. Everybody hates this word, and everybody hates cancer. Everybody! We have all lost friends and family members due to cancer. The only people that love cancer are the pharmaceutical companies. These companies make the medications to "treat" cancer. They make billions of dollars each and every year. Yes, *billions*! After years of making billions of dollars in profit for these companies, have we seen any—I repeat, *any*—significant reduction of cancer? We will walk for cancer donations, we will pledge for cancer, we will rally the troops for cancer, donating our hard-earned dollars for cancer research and treatments. Yet, Dr. John Bailer, who has been on the staff of the National Cancer Institute for the last twenty years, states, "My overall assessment, is that the national cancer programs must be judged a qualified failure."

So, how much money goes into cancer research? Well, I hope you are sitting down. According to the National Cancer Institute, our own government "funds" cancer research to the tune of about $4.9 billion dollars each year over the last six years.

Additionally, there are 260 "nonprofit" organizations dedicated to cancer "fund-raising." The big daddy in fundraising is the American Cancer Society. This organization raises over $1 billion each and every year. Of that $1 billion, about 15 percent pays for fund-raising activities, and about 60 percent of the $1 billion goes to paying salaries and benefits for the organization's employees. I'm not too impressed, either.

Now, I understand the concept of paying large salaries for high-end executives and the importance of attracting and keeping "top talent," but, in an August 2011 report from Charitywatch.org: http://bit.ly/2bJ9azACharitySalaries, American Cancer Society CEO Mr. John Seffrin has an annual salary—not including benefits—of $1,404,269. And Ms. Nancy Brown, of the American Heart Association, is paid $1,443,427. The highest-paid executive, however, is the president/CEO of Memorial Sloan-Kettering Cancer Center in New York, New York, Craig B. Thompson, MD. His annual salary is $2,925,426. They rank among the highest-paid nonprofit employees in the nation. I'm sure these CEOs are super hard workers, but that's a pretty good pay, isn't it? Makes me wonder, with salaries like that, how much they personally donate to their own "nonprofit" organizations.

Another prime example of a cancer nonprofit organization is called Susan G. Komen for the Cure, which uses the pink ribbon to raise their brand awareness and the catchphrase, "Race for the Cure" for their events. This nonprofit organization brings in around $400 million each year, yet the money that is forwarded to research is estimated at 20.9 percent, and money donated for actual treatment services is 5.6 percent. I wonder where the other 74 percent of $400 million goes?

I don't know about you, but something just doesn't seem right to me here. Even if we are willing to overlook huge salaries, benefits, lavish offices, and the actual low percentage of dollars forwarded to cancer research and treatment, there's still something that really troubles me about the billions of dollars going into cancer research. **Cancer continues to rise, and the money spent on cancer treatment and medications is also on the rise!** So, this whole "winning the War on Cancer" routine that we hear about in the media is just a fallacy.

By the way, cancer is the number two cause of death in America, and it took away my grandmother.

Heart Disease

Did you know that your heart is a muscle that works for you 24-7 and doesn't even require as much general attention as combing your hair? It literally works for you even while you are sleeping. When there a physical demand on your body or your "fight-or-flight" mechanism is activated, the heart springs into action, pumping extra blood for you. That's pretty cool. The heart, however, does not like it when you eat unhealthy foods, smoke, don't exercise, become obese, and allow yourself to become highly stressed. Taking care of your heart only requires a few simple steps to keep it running well. Some exercise, some rest, and some good nutrition—that's about it. That seems simple enough: http://bit.ly/2H7iEka10LeadingCauses.

By the way, heart disease is the number one cause of death in America.

Type 2 Diabetes

Have you heard that even our teens are now getting type 2 diabetes? Regardless of whether we are talking about a teenager or an adult, the cause will be focused around your nutrition. The amount of sugar we consume with sugar substitutes, added sugar, refined carbohydrates, junk food, candy, sodas, cake, ice cream, pie, and don't forget the alcohol, is outrageous. All of this must be broken down in our bodies and turns right into sugar or glucose in our bloodstream. Do you want to know what else leads to diabetes? Being overweight and not exercising. So, to turn your diabetes around, you have to know and understand how to eat correctly, start exercising, limit your alcohol intake, and do just a few other key items. I don't know about you, but this doesn't seem all that impossible to me. Here is a link for more information: http://wb.md/1ZVDYeR.

By the way, diabetes is the number seven cause of death.

Hospital and Medical Errors

According to the website www.hospitalsafetyscore.org, in 2013, preventable hospital and medical errors account **for approximately 440,000 American deaths each and every year.** In the peer-reviewed *Journal of Patient Safety*, Leah Binder, president and CEO, states, "We are burying a population the size of Miami every year from medical errors that can be prevented": http://bit.ly/1GxnsqD

Furthermore, a national survey showed that physicians and staff often refuse to report a serious adverse event or medical error to anyone in authority approximately 45 percent of the time (Look under **Results**). I wish I were making this up; here is the link: http://1.usa.gov/1YoGYC7. By the way, cardiologists are the highest **nonreporting** group of all specialties. So very possibly this number would be underestimated. Here are primary categories of preventable adverse events (PAEs):

- Errors of commission (first do no harm)
- Errors of omission (failure to follow guidelines)
- Errors of communication (between doctors and nurses)
- Diagnostic errors (failure to make a lifesaving diagnosis)

These medical errors have been estimated to cost our country $1 trillion each year: http://bit.ly/1UQ47YvMedicalMistakes

By the way, hospital and medical errors are estimated to be the number three cause of death.

Obesity

Obesity-related deaths include those from type 2 diabetes, hypertension, heart disease, liver disease, cancer, dementia, and depression. Nearly all have "metabolic dysfunction," as the common underlying factor. One in five American deaths are now directly associated to obesity. Obesity is known as the harbinger of death. Rarely is the actual cause of death ever reported as obesity. Instead, it is the complications that are directly due to obesity that are typically listed: cancer, heart disease, diabetes, hypertension, chronic obstructive pulmonary disease (COPD), and, according to Dr. Mercola, obesity-related diseases account for a staggering **75 percent of our health-care costs in the United States.** Check out this link: http://bit.ly/2EkQmREObesity

In my own family, we have obesity. A family member who was obese chose to have a gastric bypass procedure performed on her. Following her surgery, she had great difficulty holding down any food or even water. She saw her specialist and was told not to worry about it, be patient, and she would be fine. Just a few days later, she had a heart attack and was rushed to the emergency room. Her brain was starved of oxygen and she slipped into a coma. **She never woke from her coma and died a year later at age thirty-four.**

How Much Are We Spending?

Americans consume a lot of prescription drugs. Most commonly, drugs for cholesterol, heartburn, depression/anxiety, and especially for pain. The most recent analytics from IMS Health reveal spending on medicine increased by double digits for a second year in 2015 and that it has reached **$425 billion per year!** That's a lot of money.

The Most Profitable Medications

This is an interesting fact: **doctors who take money from drug companies prescribe more expensive drugs and procedures.** The research done by ProPublica, published in March of 2016, compiled a list of doctors and hospitals who have profited the most from direct payments from pharmaceutical and medical-device companies. A staggering $3,490,000,000 was given to doctors and hospitals during the period from August 2013 to December 2014. Leading the list, the top-paid profiting doctor is Dr. Sujata Narayan, a family medicine doctor in Stanford, California, who received an unbelievable amount of $43 million for what is termed "promotional, speaking/other." As I'm reading this on their website, I am literally stunned in disbelief. I don't know what "promotional, speaking/other," translates to, but I wished I would have studied that subject matter in college. This information is considered public knowledge if you know where to find it. Well, now you do. Here is the link: http://bit.ly/1ZN0vLcDollarsforDoctors You can input your own doctor's name in the search bar and do your own research.

OK, I'm finally getting it. It's all about the money then, right? Let's take a moment and set the stage. As a child, the media pushes unhealthy sugary cereals, juices, and sodas in their advertising. When I was a kid, if allowed, I would have eaten Kraft Macaroni & Cheese every day. This unhealthy eating just continues to get worse, because in school, you are typically served food with little nutritional value, or you may go out to eat fast food and snack on candy. Let's face it, some of us would eat candy all day every day if we could get away with it. If you are lucky enough to have parents who will cook at home, your fruits and vegetables may be bombarded with pesticides, and if we are in a hurry for dinner we will feed our family something that comes in a can or from a box. As you get older, you fill your lungs with cigarette smoke either directly or secondhand. We continue to breathe other pollutants and chemicals in the air. You are given free tap water with toxic fluoride, and the injections you receive have mercury, formaldehyde, aluminum, cortisone, and antibiotics in them: http://bit.

ly/2nUnbyxVacineIngredients With this kind of abuse to our systems, it is a wonder we live as long as we do!

Eventually, due to this style of living, our bodies start getting sick. So sick that we now need even more chemicals or prescription drugs just to be able to live or to survive. **As you might have figured out by now, the master plan is to keep you on these medications for the rest of your life.** Here is a current list of the biggest pharmaceutical money makers: http://bit.ly/2EzjZ4RDrugMoney

Lipitor: $13.5 billion per year. These are statin drugs to manage your high cholesterol.

Common Side Effects:

- Unexplained muscle pain, tenderness, or weakness
- Confusion, memory problems, dizziness
- Fever, unusual tiredness, and dark-colored urine
- Swelling, weight gain, urinating less than usual or not at all
- Increased thirst, increased urination, hunger, dry mouth, fruity breath odor, drowsiness, dry skin, blurred vision, unexplained weight loss
- Nausea, upper stomach pain, diarrhea, itching, loss of appetite, dark urine, clay-colored stools, jaundice (yellowing of the skin or eyes)
- Cough, difficulty swallowing, fever, hives, itching
- Fast heartbeat

Humira: $9.7 billion in 2012. It is known as a "biologic" and treats autoimmune diseases such as rheumatoid arthritis, Crohn's disease, psoriasis, and psoriatic arthritis. Made from Chinese hamster ovarian cells.

Common Side Effects:

- Fever, night sweats
- Weight loss, tiredness
- Nausea, stomach pain spreading to your shoulder
- Easy bruising and bleeding, pale skin

- Rapid heart rate
- Lightheadedness
- Liver problems, jaundice
- Dark urine, clay-colored stools
- Unexplained pain in your neck or back, numbness
- Headaches

Advair: $8.6 billion per year. An inhaled medication to treat asthma symptoms or chronic obstructive pulmonary disease (COPD) caused by smoking.

Common Side Effects:

- Bronchospasm (wheezing, chest tightness, trouble breathing)
- Fast or uneven heartbeat, restless feeling, tremor
- Fever, chills, stabbing chest pain, cough with yellow or green mucous
- Blurred vision, headaches, eye pain, or seeing halos around lights
- White patches or sores inside your mouth or on your lips, nausea

Plavix: $7.3 billion per year. Used to reduce the risk of heart attack or stroke. Plavix keeps platelets in the blood from coagulating, preventing blood clots in people who have already had a heart attack or stroke, or for those at high risk.

Common Side Effects:

- Nosebleed or other bleeding that will not stop
- Bloody or tarry stools, blood in your urine
- Coughing up blood or vomit that looks like coffee grounds
- Chest pain, pain spreading to the arm or shoulder, nausea, sweating, general ill feeling
- Sudden numbness or weakness, especially on one side of the body
- Sudden headache, confusion, problems with vision, speech, or balance
- Pale skin, weakness, fever, or jaundice (yellowing of the skin or eyes)

- Easy bruising, unusual bleeding (nose, mouth, vagina, or rectum), purple or red pinpoint spots under your skin

Nexium: $7.3 billion per year. For heartburn relief. Nexium is in a class of drugs called proton-pump inhibitors that reduce excessive stomach acid and treat symptoms associated with GERD or acid reflux.

Common Side Effects:

- Dizziness, confusion, headache
- Fast or uneven heart rate
- Jerking muscle movements, jittery feeling
- Fast heartbeat
- Diarrhea that is watery or bloody, nausea, gas, constipation, bloating
- Muscle cramps, muscle weakness, or limp feeling
- Cough or choking feeling, difficulty swallowing, dry mouth
- Seizure (convulsions)
- Blistering, peeling, or loosening of the skin
- Fever, hives

Seretide: $7.2 billion per year. Used for asthma and chronic obstructive pulmonary disease (COPD). This is a steroid medication.

Common Side Effects:

- Bruising from minor injury or bumps
- Difficulty speaking, hoarse voice
- Infections of the mouth or throat
- Diarrhea that is watery or bloody, nausea, gas, constipation, bloating
- Joint pain

Abilify: $6.3 billion per year. Used for antipsychotic conditions such as schizophrenia and bipolar disorder and has been heavily marketed.

Common Side Effects:

- Fever, stiff muscles, confusion, sweating, fast or uneven heartbeat
- Jerky muscle movements you cannot control
- Sudden numbness or weakness, headache, confusion or problems with vision, speech, or balance; dizziness, drowsiness
- Chills, body aches, flu symptoms, sores in your mouth and throat
- Increased thirst or urination, loss of appetite, fruity breath odor, drowsiness, dry skin, nausea, and vomiting
- Seizure (convulsions), anxiety, feeling like you might pass out
- Thoughts of hurting yourself, insomnia, weight gain
- Urinating less than usual or not at all, constipation
- Jaundice (yellowing of your skin or eyes)

Enbrel: $5.4 billion per year. Considered a "biologic," used for autoimmune conditions. This drug is made from Chinese hamster ovary cells and must be injected.

Common Side Effects:

- Redness, pain, swelling, itching at the site of injection
- Headaches
- Nausea, vomiting, diarrhea, stomach pain
- Heartburn
- Seizures
- Bruising or bleeding
- Difficulty breathing or swallowing
- Increased risk of developing serious infections, tuberculosis, lymphomas

Zyprexa: $5.3 billion per year. Used as an antipsychotic affecting your brain's chemicals to treat symptoms associated with psychotic conditions, schizophrenia, bipolar disorder, and manic depression. Is used for adults and children starting at age thirteen.

Common side effects:

- Bloating or swelling of the face, arms, hands, legs, or feet
- Change in vision, typically blurred vision
- Balance issues, walking difficulty, clumsiness, or unsteadiness
- Difficulty with swallowing
- Drooling
- Masklike face

Risperdal: $5 billion per year. Used as an antipsychotic to treat bipolar disorders and schizophrenia.

Common Side Effects:

- Increased sensitivity to temperature, heat or cold
- Easy to become dehydrated
- Impaired thinking and reactions, difficulty concentrating
- Anxiety, becoming easily agitated
- Blurred vision, difficulty moving eyes
- Decreased sexual desire or performance
- Difficulty speaking and swallowing
- Loss of balance
- Masklike face
- Memory problems

Cymbalta: $5 billion in 2012. The manufacture Eli Lilly has since lost the patent for this drug and has decreased sales since 2014. This is an antidepressant used for depression, anxiety disorder, and pain associated with neuropathy or fibromyalgia.

Common Side Effects:

- Nausea, stomach pain, loss of appetite
- Behavior or mood changes

- Dry mouth, constipation
- Fatigue and drowsiness
- Anxiety, panic attacks
- Impulsivity, irritability, agitation, hostility, aggression
- Hyperactivity, restlessness
- Increased depression
- Suicidal thoughts and hurting yourself
- Dark urine, clay-colored stools
- Hallucinations
- Headache
- Easy bruising, unusual bleeding

Crestor: $5 billion per year. This is a statin drug used for lowering cholesterol.

Common Side Effects:

- Headaches, depressed mood
- Muscle pain and weakness, joint pain
- Tiredness, fever
- Weight gain, swelling
- Increased thirst
- Confusion, memory problems
- Insomnia, nightmares
- Nausea, stomach pain, constipation
- Dark urine, clay-colored stools
- Jaundice

Seroquel: **$**4.7 billion per year. Used as an antipsychotic and alters the chemicals in your brain. Treats schizophrenia in adults and children starting at age thirteen; bipolar disorder and manic depression beginning at age ten.

Common side Effects:

- Thoughts of suicide when first taking medication
- Mood or behavior changes
- Constipation, stomach pain
- Nausea, vomiting
- Chills and cold sweats
- Dizziness, lightheadedness
- Unusual drowsiness and sleepiness
- Headaches
- Dry mouth, sore throat
- Breast swelling or discharge
- Increased appetite, weight gain

Singulair: $4.5 billion per year. Used for allergies and asthma in adults and children starting at age twelve months. Also used to prevent exercise-induced bronchospasm in adults and children starting at age six.

Common Side Effects:

- Abdominal and stomach pain
- Bloody nose
- Flu-like symptoms, general feeling of discomfort or illness
- Headache
- Joint pain
- Pain and tenderness around the eyes and cheekbones
- Shortness of breath
- Sweating
- Tightness of chest
- Difficulty swallowing
- Unusual tiredness and weakness

Aranesp: $4.4 billion per year. Used for producing red blood cells, a man-made form of a protein treating anemia, long-term kidney disease, and people receiving chemotherapy.

Common side effects:

- Heart attack, heart failure, and stroke
- Headaches, body aches
- Stomach pain
- Coughing
- Skin rash or redness
- Diarrhea
- Blood clots

Valium: I have added this "honorable mention" due to how popular this drug once was and that it was the very first drug to sell $1 billion worth of it. The Rolling Stones song referred to it as, "Mother's Little Helper." Between 1969 and 1982, Valium was the most commonly prescribed drug, with its peak use in 1978. It is not currently very profitable, since when the patent runs out the generic pill, diazepam, moves in. Used for anxiety, muscle spasms, seizures, alcohol withdrawal.

Common Side Effects:

- Memory problems
- Drowsiness, feeling tired, dizziness, spinning feeling
- Muscle weakness
- Nausea, constipation
- Blurred vision, double vision
- Loss of sexual desire
- Drooling or dry mouth, slurred speech

Making Money from Addiction

Here are twenty-one facts on America's Big-Pharma nightmare from Global Research by Michael Snyder: http://bit.ly/2gQ6Bt6AddictionMoney

Has there ever been a nation more hooked on drugs than the United States? And I am not just talking about illegal drugs—the truth is that the number of Americans addicted to legal drugs is far greater than the number of Americans addicted to illegal drugs. As you will read about below, more than 30 million Americans are currently on antidepressants, and doctors in the United States wrote more than 250 million prescriptions for painkillers last year. Sadly, most people get hooked on these drugs very innocently. They trusted their doctors would never prescribe something for them that would be harmful, and they trusted that the federal government would never approve any drugs that were not safe. And once the drug companies get you hooked, they often have you for life. You see, the reality of the matter is that some of these "legal drugs" are actually some of the most addictive substances on the entire planet. And when they start raising the prices on those drugs, there isn't much that the addicts can do about it. It is a brutally efficient business model, and the pharmaceutical industry guards their territory fiercely. Very powerful people will often do some really crazy things when there are hundreds of billions of dollars at stake. The following are twenty-one facts about America's endless pharmaceutical nightmare that *everyone* should know...

1. According to the *New York Times*, more than 30 million Americans are currently taking antidepressants.
2. The rate of antidepressant use among middle-aged women is far higher than for the population as a whole. One out of every four women in their forties and fifties is taking an antidepressant medication.
3. Americans account for about 5 percent of the global population, but we buy more than 50 percent of the pharmaceutical drugs.
4. Americans also consume a whopping 80 percent of all prescription painkillers.
5. It is hard to believe, but doctors in the United States write 259 million prescriptions for painkillers each year. Prescription painkillers are

some of the most addictive legal drugs, and our doctors are serving as enablers for millions upon millions of Americans who find themselves hooked on drugs.

6. Overall, pharmaceutical drug use in America is at an all-time high. According to a study conducted by the Mayo Clinic, nearly 70 percent of all Americans are on at least one prescription drug, and 20 percent of all Americans are on at least five prescription drugs.
7. According to the CDC, approximately nine out of every ten Americans who are at least sixty years old say that they have taken at least one prescription drug within the last month.
8. In 2010, the average teen in the United States was taking 1.2 central-nervous-system-type drugs. Those are the kind of drugs that treat conditions such as ADHD and depression.
9. A very disturbing Government Accountability Office report found that approximately one-third of all foster children in the United States are on at least one psychiatric drug.
10. An astounding 95 percent of the "experimental medicines" that the pharmaceutical industry produces are found not to be safe and are never approved. Of the remaining 5 percent that are approved, we often do not find out all of the toxic side effects and addictive qualities until decades later.
11. One study discovered that mothers who took antidepressants during pregnancy were four times more likely to have a baby who developed an autism spectrum disorder.
12. It has been estimated that prescription drugs kill approximately 200,000 people in the United States every single year.
13. An American will die from an unintentional prescription drug overdose every nineteen minutes. According to Dr. Sanjay Gupta, accidental prescription drug overdose is "the leading cause of acute preventable death for Americans."
14. In the United States today, prescription painkillers kill more Americans than heroin and cocaine combined.
15. According to the CDC, approximately three-quarters of a million people a year are rushed to emergency rooms in the United States because of adverse reactions to pharmaceutical drugs.

16. The number of prescription-drug-overdose deaths in the United States is five times higher than it was back in 1980.
17. A survey conducted for the National Institute on Drug Abuse found that more than 15 percent of all US high school seniors abuse prescription drugs.
18. More than twenty-six million women over the age of twenty-five say that they are using prescription medication for "unintended uses."
19. If all of these antidepressants are helping, then why are more Americans killing themselves? The suicide rate for Americans between the ages of thirty-five and sixty-four increased by nearly 30 percent between 1999 and 2010. The number of Americans who die by suicide is now greater than the number of Americans who die because of car accidents every year.
20. Antidepressant use has been linked to mass shootings in America over and over and over again, and yet the mainstream media is very quiet about this. Is it because they don't want to threaten one of their greatest sources of advertising revenue?
21. The amount of money that the pharmaceutical industry is raking in is astronomical. Americans spent $465 billion on prescription drugs during 2015 alone.

If these drugs were not so addictive and designed by the pharmaceutical companies for you to stay on them for life, they would make a lot less money. All research points to the pharmaceutical companies being primarily focused on making money!

Are you starting to figure out that these all-too-common diseases that we live with are mostly brought on by our lifestyle? And to a degree, our unwillingness to change our habits? The good news is that you can actually do something about this by educating yourself. You can actually turn your health around. If you decide to get serious about your health, reach out to our office and schedule a consultation with me. I love helping people with their health.

The next chapter is on sugar and junk food. I believe these are the gateway drugs leading into poor health habits. Once compounded, your health continues a downward spiral. You can make the changes; I know you can! First, read chapter 3.

Sugar and Junk Food, the Real Gateway Drugs

Almost everybody loves sugar, don't they? There is even a cute little name for it: "a sweet tooth." C'mon, that sounds pretty harmless, doesn't it? For the record, sugar is one of the most addictive ingredients in the world today! Today's sugars are very refined and concentrated more than ever before. It's estimated that the average American consumes anywhere from a one-quarter to one-half a pound of sugar per day. Consuming sugar in these amounts can lead to similar symptoms to a drug addiction; dependence, cravings, and withdrawal. The good news is that we can train our taste buds to accept less sugar. I have personally spent three years breaking my sugar addiction.

The turning point for me was that my cousin had recently died from pancreatic cancer. The pancreas is the organ that secretes insulin in our body. When we consume lots of sugar we are putting heavy demands on our pancreas. The three primary things that lead to pancreatic cancer are excess sugar/fructose consumption, lack of exercise, and lack of vitamin D.

An article from *The American Journal of Clinical Nutrition* states that "high consumption of sugar and sugar sweetened foods increases the risk of pancreatic cancer." For more information, go to: http://bit.ly/1rp1Z2hSugar-Cancer

As a doctor, I am able to research and understand this quite easily, and I decided it was high time to make the changes. The first thing I did was I made myself a deal. I would not personally buy any candy anymore, period. I just wouldn't buy it. I did pretty good with that but the addiction continued. My favorite sugary sweet, my go-to candy was Peanut M&Ms. I loved, loved, loved them! It got so bad that if I was visiting you, and by chance you would have a bowl of M&Ms sitting out, I would pray you wouldn't turn your back on me because they would be gone! After embarrassing myself on a handful of occasions, I decided that behavior needed to stop. I just stopped eating all chocolate and candy. Was it hard to do? You bet!

I found an immediate replacement food though: fruit. I'm not talking a few pieces per day. I'm talking fruit all day long! The sugar in fruit, called fructose, is obviously way better than refined sugar, and certainly fruit contains fiber and lots of nutrients that are great for your body too. However, fructose is broken down in the liver and leads to increasing levels of uric acid (which can cause gout), fat around your midline, and increases your blood levels of lipids. Bottom line here, I'm still addicted! Weaning myself down from excessive fruit consumption was a much easier than from refined sugar. There were some additional organic products that I used that were very helpful for me in releasing the final grips of that sugar addiction. I've been free from the addiction to sugar for about three years now, and I've been slowly reintroducing certain fruits that are organic with a low glycemic index and in much smaller quantities.

Added Sugars

When you read a label and it says, "added sugar," it is not the sugar that is naturally found in fruits. It means it is an added amount to the processed food. The high level of added sugar changes our brain chemistry to cause binging, cravings, withdrawal symptoms, and sensitization. Excessive sugar can change the neural pathways in the brain, just like the addiction to drugs or alcohol. In fact, sugar addiction can be even harder habit to break because it also affects our bodies' stress hormones. Stories in the press about Oreos being more addictive than cocaine may have been overstated and somewhat funny. However, rest assured that the power of sugar will lure us in again and again and eventually will steal our health from us.

The drug analogy is always a tough one because, unlike drugs, food is necessary for survival. However, research shows that sugar stimulates the reward-processing center in the brain the same way that drug abuse does. This translates into an actual addiction to sugary foods.

Sugar is rarely consumed by itself; for example, by the spoonful. It is typically combined with artificial flavorings (soda), or with fat and starch (cakes and muffins), which results in combinations that send the brain's pleasure centers into overdrive—which is why it is *no surprise* that so many of us are addicted to sugar. This is one fascinating area of scientific research that I hope continues. One thing is very clear: sugar, no matter the form—agave, white sugar, brown sugar, coconut nectar, honey, and fruit—is everywhere, and we are consuming way too much of it.

Sugar Is Slowly Killing Us

What is so interesting about sugar is that it is socially acceptable and often considered "a treat," when it really should be thought of as "toxic poison." Research shows that sugar can be more addicting than cocaine, activating the opiate receptors in our brain and affecting our brains' reward centers. This can lead to compulsive behavior, despite the negative consequences; for example, weight gain, headaches, hormone imbalances, cavities, diabetes, increased cancer risk, obesity, raised cholesterol, and heart disease. Studies reveal that every time we eat sweets we are reinforcing those neural pathways causing the brain to become increasingly hardwired to crave sugar, building up a tolerance like any other drug. It also provokes similar withdrawal symptoms once you're addicted. On the outside sugar seems pretty harmless, but on the inside, it is killing us. Once you're addicted, it can be a very difficult (and for some, impossible) addiction to beat. Here is an interesting link from WebMD: http://bit.ly/2G6pN34AddictivePoison

Our Bodies Were Not Designed for This Much Sugar

I don't like using the word *addiction* when it comes to food. When you have an addiction to alcohol or drugs, it's recommended to avoid them completely. Food is different. You need food to survive, and I think it's unrealistic to think you will be able to completely quit sugar. That being said, there are many studies that show our brains respond to sugar in a similar way that it does to illicit and addictive drugs. The problem is, we weren't meant to enjoy sugars and sweeteners in such highly concentrated amounts. In nature, sugar is found surrounded by fiber; for example, in sugarcane and in fruits. In nature, it comes in that natural fiber container that produces a shorter blood-sugar response and aids in fullness. The natural sugar in fruit is called fructose, and we must limit the amount of consumption of fruit as well. Even though fruit is natural, it is in fact still sugar according to your body.

Fructose needs to be digested by the liver and triggers the formation of lipogenesis (the production of fats like triglycerides and cholesterol), uric acid, and free radicals. Worse yet is the chemical sweetener called high-fructose corn syrup (HFCS). In higher doses it can rot holes in your intestinal lining. It is known to trigger the inflammation in our body that we know is at the root of obesity, diabetes, cancer, heart disease, dementia, and accelerated aging. Do yourself and your family a huge favor and stay away from anything with high-fructose corn syrup!

The Chemical Sweetener Aspartame

Aspartame is the artificial and neurotoxic sweetener that is found in almost everything that says "diet" or "sugar-free." Aspartame, which is commonly used in diet soda, is **two hundred times sweeter than natural sugar, is addictive, and is a toxin to our nervous system**. Additionally, it has many side effects. In a recent study conducted by researchers from the University of Miami Miller School of Medicine and at Columbia University Medical Center, it was discovered that those who drank diet soda drinks on a daily basis were more likely to contract vascular diseases compared to those who did not drink diet drinks with aspartame. Furthermore, the diet soda drinkers had a 70 percent increase in waist size than those who did not drink them. If this study doesn't open your eyes, I seriously don't know what will. I recommend this link to learn more: http://bit.ly/2Epm1FCAspartameAddiction

Ten Similarities of Sugar, Junk Food, and Abusive Drugs

There are many ridiculous myths in nutrition. The idea that losing weight is all about calories and willpower is one of the worst. The truth is that sugar and highly processed junk foods can be addictive, just like drugs, influencing our behavioral symptoms and our actions too. This translates into cravings. Here are ten disturbing similarities between sugar, junk food, and abusive drugs:

1. Junk Foods Flood the Brain with Dopamine

Our brains are hardwired to want to perform certain behaviors. Mostly, these are behaviors that are important for our survival, such as eating. When we eat, a brain hormone called dopamine is released into an area of the brain called the reward center. We interpret this dopamine signal as "pleasure." This will program our brain to make us want to do that behavior over and over again. This is one of the ways the brain evolved to help us navigate through our natural environment, motivating us to do things that helped our species to thrive and survive. This is considered a good thing, because without dopamine, our lives would be boring and miserable.

The problem is that in our modern world, we have substances that are now considered "superstimuli," which will **flood our brains with dopamine**—way more than we were ever exposed to throughout evolution. This leads to our brain pathways being "hijacked" by the intense dopamine signal. A great example of this is the drug cocaine. When people take cocaine, it floods the brain with dopamine, and the brain changes its programming to want more cocaine again and again and again. The dopamine pathways that are supposed to guide people toward survival have now been taken over by this new "stimulus," which releases more dopamine and is a much stronger behavioral reinforcer than anything we have in the natural environment.

From a scientific point of view, this is where it gets interesting. Sugar and highly processed junk foods have been proven to have the same effect as drugs of abuse. Here is where you can learn more: http://1.usa.gov/1TVK9xJ

Junk food and sugar floods our brain with dopamine and directly affects our brains' reward centers. Sugar also has some effects on opioid pathways within the brain; this is the same system that is used by drugs like heroin and morphine! This is why highly processed, sugar-laden foods can make some people lose control over their consumption; they literally hijack their brain pathways just like drugs will, leading to overeating.

Bottom Line: Studies have shown that sugar and junk foods literally flood the reward center in the brain with dopamine, stimulating the same areas as drugs of abuse like cocaine, heroin, and morphine. This results in dependence and overconsumption.

2. Junk Foods Can Lead to Powerful Cravings

Cravings can be a very powerful feeling. People often confuse cravings with hunger, but the two are *not* the same. Hunger is caused by various complex physiological signals that involve the body's need for energy and desire for nutrients. However, people often get cravings despite having just finished a fulfilling, nutritious meal.

This is because cravings are not always about satisfying your body's need for energy. Instead, they are your brain calling for a reward. In other words, your brain drives you toward that dopamine/opioid pleasure signal, which is not natural and has nothing to do with real hunger. These types of craving for junk foods are very similar to cravings for drugs, cigarettes, and other addictive substances. The obsessive nature and thought processes of addicts are identical.

Bottom Line: Cravings are a common symptom when it comes to both junk foods and addictive drugs and have very little to do with actual hunger. This is much more than just a self-control issue.

3. Imaging Studies of the Brain

Tracking brain functions is accomplished with MRI scans. These scans reveal changes in blood flow, which is directly tied to the activation of neurons. Using a MRI scan will show that both food and drugs can activate the same brain regions when people crave either junk food or drugs.

Bottom Line: Scientists use MRI scans to show that the same brain regions are activated in response to cravings for both junk food and drugs.

4. A Tolerance Builds Up to Our Reward Centers

When the brain gets flooded with dopamine, a protective mechanism begins. The brain starts reducing its number of dopamine receptors in order to keep things balanced. The scientific word for this is "downregulation." This is a fancy word for building up tolerance. This is a well-known feature of drug abuse. People need progressively larger and larger doses because the brain reduces its number of receptors for the "pleasurable" experience. The same applies to junk food. This is the reason why food addicts will sometimes eat huge amounts in a single sitting. As the brain receptors have built up a tolerance they will need more to become satisfied. Building up tolerance is one of the hallmarks of addiction. It is common to all forms of drug and alcohol abuse and also applies to sugar and junk food as well. This is an excellent link to learn more: http://bit.ly/2G9AxOdSugarAddiction

Bottom Line: When the brain's reward system is repeatedly overstimulated, it responds by reducing its number of pleasure receptors. This leads to an increase in tolerance, which is one of the hallmarks of addiction.

5. Many People Binge on Junk Foods

When addicts become increasingly tolerant to the effects of a drug, they start increasing the dosage. Instead of one pill, they take two, then three, then four, or even ten. Because there are now fewer receptors in the brain, a larger dose is needed to reach the same effect. This is the reason why some people binge on junk food. Binge eating is a well-known feature of food addiction as well as other eating disorders that share common symptoms with drug abuse. There are also numerous studies in rats showing that they will binge on junk food just like they would binge on addictive drugs.

Bottom Line: Binge eating is a common symptom of food addiction. It is caused by an increasing tolerance, making the brain need a larger dose than before to reach the same pleasurable effects.

6. Cross-Sensitization: Lab Animals Can Switch from Drugs to Sugar and Vice Versa

Cross-sensitization is one feature of addictive substances. It involves being able to "switch" easily from one addiction to another. Studies have shown that lab animals who have become dependent on sugar can easily switch to amphetamines or cocaine. This fact is another strong argument for the case that sugar, and junk food can become addictive.

Bottom Line: Studies show that addicted rats can switch between sugar, amphetamine, and cocaine. This, "cross-sensitization" is another hallmark of addictive substances.

7. Drugs That Fight Addiction Are Now Being Prescribed for Weight Loss!

Does this really seem like a good idea prescribing yet another medication? Another argument for the addictive nature of junk food is that the same drugs used to fight drug addiction are now being used to help people lose weight and fight food addiction. The fact that the same types of drugs can help people eat fewer calories and lose weight implies that food addiction shares some of the same biological and neural pathways as addiction to narcotics.

Bottom Line: Drugs that have been used to fight addictions such as smoking, alcoholism, and heroin are now being used for weight loss. This indicates that food affects the brain in similar ways as these drugs of abuse.

8. Abstaining Can Lead to Withdrawal Symptoms

Withdrawal symptoms are another key feature of addiction. This is when addicted individuals experience adverse symptoms when they stop ingesting the substance they are addicted to. A prominent example is caffeine withdrawal. A lot of people who are addicted to caffeine get headaches, feel tired, and become irritable if they abstain from coffee for long periods of time. In the lab, rats who are made dependent on sugar experience clear withdrawal symptoms when the sugar is removed. These symptoms include teeth chattering, head shakes, and forepaw tremors, like the withdrawal symptoms experienced from opiate addiction.

Bottom Line: There is plenty of evidence that abstaining from sugar and junk food can lead to clear withdrawal-type symptoms.

9. Junk Foods Are Seriously Harmful to Physical Health

Junk foods are unhealthy, and there is no doubt about it. They have excessive amounts of harmful ingredients like sugar, refined wheat, and refined oils. At the same time, they contain very low amounts of healthy ingredients like fiber, protein, and micronutrients. Not only do junk foods make people eat more than they're supposed to, but the ingredients in them can be directly linked to cancer, heart disease, obesity, metabolic syndrome and type 2 diabetes.

This is not a controversial subject anymore. It is basic common knowledge. Everyone knows that junk food is unhealthy. Even with this knowledge, they still eat junk food in excessive quantities, despite knowing better. This is also common with drug abuse and addiction. Addicts know that the drugs are causing them physical harm, but they take them anyway.

Bottom Line: It is common knowledge that junk foods are harmful, but many people are still unable to control their consumption.

10. Food Addiction Symptoms and the Medical Diagnosis for Addiction

There is no easy way of measuring addiction. There is no blood test, breathalyzer, or urine test that can determine if someone is addicted. Instead, the diagnosis is based on a set of **behavioral symptoms**. If you look at the criteria for a substance use disorder, you will see the resemblance to food-related behaviors. For example, being unable to "cut back" on your eating despite wanting to. Also, cravings and urges to use the substance and continuing to use despite physical problems that occur, such as weight gain. Any of this sound familiar? These are classic symptoms of addiction. You can learn more here: http://bit.ly/2EZxOYhAddictionSymptoms

Bottom Line: The truth of the matter is, there is no fundamental difference between junk food addiction and drug addiction. It's just a different substance of abuse, and the social consequences aren't as severe. I have spoken to former addicts who have also had problems with sugar and junk food. They agree that the symptoms are not just similar, but downright identical.

If you need help getting off the sugar, the sweeteners, or the junk food, I suggest that you reach out to our office and schedule a consultation with me.

The next chapter on "Reclaiming Your Body" will get you focused on your attitude, self-image, having fun, and being good to yourself. We also begin to talk about nutrition and exercise.

Reclaiming Your Body

Are you happy with the way you look? Are we *ever* happy with the way we look? By a show of hands, is there any of us who doesn't want to improve the way we look, our self-image, or our sex appeal? Exactly what I thought. Everybody wants to look better and feel better about themselves. And that translates into wanting to look better to others too. We have been beating ourselves up since we were kids about the way we look. We all do it. I have always thought we should be our own best cheerleaders! Let's face it, no one is perfect, and we are never going to be perfect. Thank God we can give up that fantasy!

Can You Get Your Body Back?

I absolutely believe you can. It is easy to read a nice article and feel good about yourself for a few minutes. But later, reality will again hit you with the truth. To make physical changes with your body, you will need to get to work. Not only will it take work, it will take time too. Almost daily, I see advertisements for quick and easy weight loss with no exercise needed. Are you kidding me? Six-pack abs with no exercise, really? Lose fifty pounds in three weeks, really? I've never been a fan of lying to myself or to anyone else for that matter! It's true, part of feeling good about yourself is in your mind. The other part is with your body. The great news is you don't have to have a perfect hourglass figure or have six-pack abs. I believe as long as you are working on it and getting results, you will naturally start feeling good about yourself. These results can't be overstated. I know plenty of people who work out and go to the gym but never get results. How frustrating! To me, that is simply wasting your time. Yes, you are at least doing something positive for yourself; however, when you are getting results, well, that is where the magic is!

As we all know, the mind communicates with the body, and the body communicates with the mind; it is the effort that you put in that is the key. In our own minds, we *know* whether or not we are putting in the effort. I remember that as a child in elementary school I would get a little sticky star on my shirt for putting in the effort. Thinking back, I would put in a lot of effort for those little sticky stars! We know inside our own heads that the self-confidence in putting in the work (effort) is much different than copying another kid's school work. I suggest if you really want to make the changes, feeling good and looking good and really improving your health, you need to have your "whys" in place first. Think. Just think about why it is important to you. How will it benefit your family and their health? Because we will all hit a few stumbling blocks along the way. At times, life always will get in the way. I can guarantee you one thing, though: putting in the work will always give you your self-confidence and your sex-appeal back every time!

In Scott Haltzman, MD's book, *The Secrets of Happily Married Women*, he says, "One of the main reasons I've found that women don't want to have sex is that they don't feel as sexy as they used to." Unfortunately, feeling sexy isn't something you can just conjure up at a moment's notice. "Women, have to transition between the mother who's taking care of everything to the seductive wife, and that doesn't happen in an instant. It takes work."

Us guys have our issues too. As we all know by now, our testosterone declines as we mature; that is a fact. Poor nutrition habits will certainly not help. Smoking will ruin your circulation, and without circulation and excellent blood flow to...certain areas...well, you know. Drinking certainly doesn't help. Lack of exercise doesn't improve blood flow or circulation. Medications are absolutely full of side effects and more than likely decrease our interest and performance. Coupled with a lack of sleep, stress, responsibilities, and overeating, well, let's just say, we may not feel like Rudolph Valentino 24-7, either.

Your Attitude

Why your attitude? I will tell you why: it's because this is all about you! Your attitude about yourself, your attitude about others, and your attitude about your self-image will have a lot to do with the way you connect with others—and your family too. So, do yourself a big favor and keep yours in check, especially around the people in your life who you truly care about. A good attitude will help with your self-image as well. Funny how it just feeds right back around again!

Here are three steps to getting your sexy back that you might want to take into consideration:

1. **Flirt, communicate, and be interesting:** Learn to flirt! People who are self-assured and comfortable are rare. Make yourself stand out by being unafraid to make a move. Take initiative in conversations, speak clearly and confidently, and let the other person know you're interested. You don't have to be drop-dead handsome, a swimsuit model, or a genius to be good at talking to people or flirting. All it takes is some self-assurance, a little bit of courage, and thinking about the other person instead of yourself. You can become more interesting and even irresistible if you are willing to put yourself out there just a little bit. I believe this is especially important when in a long-term relationship or marriage. And, just so that there is clarity with this, I am suggesting flirting with your mate!
2. **Make yourself feel good:** Whether you're going out for a night on the town, hanging out with your spouse, or just running errands, if you want to "up" your sex appeal, make your own comfort and confidence a priority. For some of us, that might mean rocking a new pair of pumps and a tight-fitting dress. For others, you may feel more confident in a straightforward shirt or well-fitting pants. Whatever you're wearing, if you feel good about yourself that will always help your self-image. Try to find some middle ground between the "sweatpants-and-slippers" level of comfort and the "six-inch-Louboutins" level of supersexy high fashion. You don't need to have a tuxedo on to look great, but you do need to make sure your clothes are appropriately fitting, clean, and that you are well groomed and looking your best if you want to step up your self-confidence and attitude.
3. **Take care of your body:** Spend a little time each day grooming yourself and giving your body the care and attention, it needs and deserves. Hair, makeup, oral hygiene, and other little things can do wonders for

your self-confidence. Be sure to smell good while you are at it. Be confident that you've done everything necessary to look your best. For us guys, nose hair, ear hair, and eyebrows are important. I really can't explain why the overgrowth of ear and nose hair occurs as we mature, but it does. I have known many guys who just seem to love their crazy eyebrow hair that grows wild. Hey, if this turns your gal on, then keep 'em growin' and "get 'er done!"

Perfection

Please just stop. Stop striving for the perfect this or the perfect that. Let's just say for the sake of argument that it simply is not going to happen, ever! The truth of the matter is that even swimsuit models and exotic or Chippendale dancers don't have perfect bodies, at least in their own minds. Bodybuilders are typically the same way. Professional pictures that we see are typically altered, airbrushed, with tons of makeup and lighting. So we need to get perfection completely out of our minds or we are setting ourselves up for failure, and that is not what we are about.

Long ago, I learned to swap out the word *perfection* for the word *excellence*. What this does is it takes all the pressure off being perfect, and you simply strive for excellence. This was a small distinction in my own mind that I changed many years ago, and what a difference it made. There will always be someone better looking, someone faster, someone taller, someone with better hair, longer legs, and so on. I still have a few "issues" with perfection from time to time; however, as I mature, it gets easier and easier to let go.

Reality

You do not have to have a chiseled, hard body to gain more confidence and pride in your appearance. If, however, you don't feel comfortable with your arms, stomach, thighs, or some other part of your body, then simply work on it! I will always go back to the fact that you have to put the work in to your body to get fit. This is what it takes to get in better shape, and it helps you become more confident with your body. Let's face it, even losing a few pounds can begin this process, and that can have an enormous effect on your self-confidence and self-image.

I realize that we not only expect but demand fast results. We have been conditioned to believe it can all happen overnight, or your "money back." The truth is, it typically takes many years to finally wake up to the reality that our health has gone to hell, our energy is completely in the tank, and with that, our attitude has usually become quite stinky as well. So what are we going to do about this? If you are in a position to stop everything and immerse yourself in a six-month all-inclusive "boot camp," without any distractions or responsibilities that promises to cure everything that ails you, well congrats. You are in a very special place, and I'm quite sure that you will have great results—and frankly, I would like to join you! For most of us, though, we will have to at least get started and then stay consistent, and the results, I promise you, will come.

It seems as we mature, our responsibilities grow, and let's face it, these responsibilities literally take up most of our day. By nightfall we are frequently out of energy and too tired to exercise or even cook a healthy meal, let alone prepare our meals for the next day. So, we sit around, relax, read a good book, watch some TV. Before long, we are asleep in the chair. The problem with this is that we need to change our habits, or we will never get started.

I always recommend starting slow, learning the basics, and building good healthy habits that will build on your future. It is with these good habits and consistency that you will get the results you are looking for. Without learning the basics first, I can guarantee you that somewhere in your future, life will get in the way and you will at some point become derailed from your program. This is exactly why having the basics down and having your systems in place is vital for long-term success with your health.

We all have issues whether they are mental, emotional, or physical. Overcoming these and working around them is always going to be my recommendation. I believe that while you are putting in the work, you will find these issues becomes less and less of an issue. As you continue moving forward, with your system in place, it helps to keep you on track each and every day.

Reclaiming Your Body

"How to Get Your Sexy Back" from *Redbook* magazine reveals twenty-one recommendations that will benefit you in many ways by improving your self-confidence, friendship, and communication with your friends and family: http://wb.md/1n0G8GC

1. Focus on a prior experience.

Take a few minutes out of your busy day to replay a romantic encounter with your mate, how that made you feel, and how exciting that was is a powerful technique.

2. Pamper yourself.

Take the time after the long hot shower to massage your body with some lotion. Use the massager on your shower head to give yourself a relaxing and therapeutic neck massage. Some people enjoy using a soft skin brush in the shower as part of the routine.

3. Watch a romantic movie with a little steam.

Sometimes relaxing and watching a romantic movie can do wonders. Especially if it is a little "steamy." Women are visual creatures (just like men), and when you give your eyes a sensual treat, it can build some romance and set the mood.

4. Throw away the Victoria's Secret catalog.

Comparing yourself to unrealistic body ideals is a surefire way to feel unsexy. Remove these images from your life as much as you possibly can (as in, turn off *The Bachelor* and all those size zero bikini bodies). Remind yourself that you are on your journey now and that you are working on it, staying focused on results. Relax; you will get there.

5. Ditch the sweats.

"If sweats have become your standard after-work uniform, then you are unlikely to feel sexy," says Sari Locker, the author of *The Complete Idiot's Guide* to Amazing Sex. You don't have to wear fishnets, but "buy some clothes that make you feel sexy when you're lounging, even if it's just a silky camisole and leggings." When you look and feel appealing to your mate, you will probably look and feel appealing to your mate!

6. Get away.

Take a walk or plan a girls' or a guys' night out. When you do something just for yourself, it's easier to remember who you were before you acquired all of your responsibilities in life. I've always believed spending time with friends can help us feel more balanced and happier overall.

7. Exercise.

There are reasons to exercise and to hit the gym. Losing weight and lowering stress are two easy ones. But the best one is to boost your sexiness. Sweat releases endorphins, giving you a natural high. If you are feeling low, then go hit the gym, go for a walk, or go ride your bike. Start moving; you will feel stronger, and your attitude should immediately improve. Additionally, having muscle tone is always sexy.

8. Get nostalgic.

Create your favorite playlists that remind you of when you were falling in love with your husband or wife. Sometimes just hearing those tunes can send thoughts to when you were falling in love. You can take out old photos from when you two crazy kids first started dating. When you go out together, talk about some of the more "interesting" experiences you may have had, back in the day. The conversation may be well received.

9. Make your best feature pop.

Play up your eyes with a new eyeliner or try a different gloss on your lips. "When you feel beautiful, you feel sensual," says Debbie Mandel, the author of *Turn On Your Inner Light*. Take a few extra minutes to primp yourself and feel pretty. If you are a guy and you have good arms, then make sure your shirt fits you in a way to show them off.

10. Buy new underthings.

Throw away those ripped, faded, you've-had-them-for-four-years underwear. Guys, we know that we wear our underwear way too long. Do something about that.

11. Stop worrying.

When you're focused on worry, the last thing on your mind is feeling sexy, says Louann Brizendine, the author of *The Female Brain,* http://bit.ly/2nWQd0kFemaleBrain and *The Male Brain,* http://bit.ly/2o1qVNSMaleBrain, try to pinpoint what's bothering you and try to set it aside. Write down your concerns and tuck them away. And, for Pete's sake, stop stressing over your thighs or your tummy pooch. He is going to be much more interested in how interesting you are than anything else.

12. Breathe.

Mindful breaths enhance and reinforce the mind-body connection. For a few minutes each morning, close your eyes and breathe deeply. Clear your thoughts and focus on being calm. When you're relaxed, it's easier to get in touch with your inner self.

13. Look in the mirror.

From the onset of puberty, we're taught to scrutinize every imperfection of our body. Instead, give yourself a reaffirming reality check by doing just the opposite. Go ahead, give yourself a compliment; I dare you!

14. Turn off the phone.

And the TV, and your laptop. Life's distractions keep you from being fully in touch with yourself and your loved ones. Unplug so you can plug in to what's important: you. Focus on just one activity, like reading a book or listening to a podcast. You can journal your thoughts or focus on your goals. Tuning out the world helps make you the priority, which in turn reminds you just how lovable you are.

15. Move your body.
Not a good dancer? Fake it! Turn on your favorite tunes and just let go. Move your entire body to the beat. For us guys, play the "air guitar," or that favorite drum solo that you love—you know the one. It felt good then, and it will feel good now.

16. Create a kid-free zone.
Nothing kills sensuality like a room full of Tinker Toys, diaper bags, and crayon-drawn art. Have a space in your house that's adult-only so you can focus on yourselves. It has been suggested to make your bedroom that place. No children's toys, no pictures of adorable faces; it is the environment for Mom and Dad.

17. Change it up.
Take an art class. Or book a last-minute weekend getaway. Novelty is the greatest aphrodisiac, and by switching up your routine you can create spontaneity. Doing something out of the ordinary creates excitement in your life. Excitement is *always* fun, and we should do it more often.

18. Hit the spa.
Get a manicure, pedicure, bikini wax, or massage! Taking care of yourself boosts your confidence and reminds you that you are worth it.

19. Illuminate your nights.
Light a scented candle in your den or break out those candlesticks for dinner. Candlelight casts a warm, cozy glow over everything and everyone in

the room and is so much more flattering than harsh light bulbs. You will literally and figuratively see yourself in a new light. Guys, always set the mood with the lighting whenever possible, and while you are at it, set the music too!

20. Strike a pose.

A recent study in the *Journal of Sexual Medicine* found that women who regularly practiced yoga felt sexier. Researchers say it could be because yoga forges a stronger mind-body connection through meditation and creates self-confidence, which can lead to feeling more romantic. I would believe this will work for us men also.

21. Create a bathing ritual.

Once a week (or more, if you're lucky), light candles, run a bath, add a foaming bath gel, and submerge yourself in a warm tub. "Sure, it's a cliché," says Elizabeth Lombardo, PhD, the author of *A Happy You: Your Ultimate Prescription for Happiness*. "But it works." There's nothing like warm suds on your naked body to pump up the sensuality factor and remind you how important it is to take time to reconnect with yourself. So what are you waiting for? Go fill up the tub. In my case, I'll jump in the hot tub!

Take Some Action

If you want your body to physically change, riding a bicycle or walking on the treadmill will certainly help, and it is a great start. But if you want serious change with your body it will take much more than that. You know, and I know that you will need to "get to work" if you really want to reclaim your body! Here are some basics:

- Lift weights; it's the fastest, most efficient way to change your body shape.
- Do intervals, the most efficient way to burn calories.
- Practice sprints and work your lower body.
- Get some vitamin D.

- Increase dietary fat like avocados, coconut oil, fish, nuts.
- Take your vitamins, minerals, and superfoods.
- Prioritize rest; get a minimum of seven hours each night.
- Eat more protein, including eggs.
- Do squats and take shorter rest periods.
- Resistance training builds muscle, increases metabolism, and burns calories.
- Don't drink (much).
- Don't smoke.

We have created many programs and systems in our office to help you reclaim your body; the one that is right for you is dependent on your goals, your physical ability, and your willingness to exercise. This includes support groups to help you achieve your goals. Call our office for a consultation if you are serious!

In the next chapter, "Feeding Your Mind," we go even deeper into the importance of having that ever-elusive "peace of mind," learning to relax, and not taking yourself so darn seriously!

PART II

The Solutions That You Can Use

Relaxing Your Mind

We love our distractions, and sometimes we get wrapped up and almost attracted to the drama, don't we? First, let's talk about what distractions really are. In today's world, we can get distracted literally in a heartbeat. Distractions are caused by our lack of ability to pay attention, or simply a lack of interest, period. Distractions come from both external sources and internal sources. External distractions can be from visual triggers, social interactions, music, what's on TV, text messages, phone calls; the list goes on and on. The internal distractions come from hunger, fatigue, illness, worrying, and daydreaming. Both external and internal distractions will interfere with your focus and lead to a short attention span.

Many times, we seem to pride ourselves on our ability to multitask, literally juggling numerous projects, people, and conversations at once. It is noted that women have a better ability to multitask than men. Regardless, if true or not, does that really keep you and your mind happy? Does that give us peace and tranquility? Do we seem to sleep better at night when we are constantly problem solving the multitude of projects and people and family problems? More importantly, are we really more present with our loved ones when we are multitasking? I don't think so.

The Art of Distraction

Contemporary life is full of distractions; phone calls, e-mails, and texts; political banter; Facebook discussions about cats, dogs, and dress colors; TV shows; and whatever the latest viral video craze is. A magician is the consummate professional at the art of distraction. Shiny objects certainly distract our attention: new cars, new toys, new outfits, new shoes, football season. It has become an expectation that you are and must stay connected. We seem to think our friends are following and paying attention to our social media posts too. I have personally used the words, "didn't you see my Facebook post?" Once I realized what I had asked, I wished I hadn't. Increasingly, we seem to be more and more expected to be more and more connected. But does all that "noise" make us happy?

Let's say you woke up one day and decided you no longer wanted to participate in this Age of Distraction. Do you think you could just drop out and unplug? Well, you could, but you'd be up against an entire culture that expects you to constantly participate. My good friend recently did just that: completely unplugged. I am sorry to say that I actually tried to stop him. "How could you possibly do that?" I asked. He responded with, "Watch me." Last I heard, he was basking on a warm beach in an undisclosed location. He says he is peaceful and enjoying "the life." Once he is completely settled in, I'm going to visit, just to make sure.

Minimize Distractions for a Happier Mind

Managing your work environment and minimizing distractions certainly helps you get more done. How often are you distracted at work or at home? What a crazy question, right? Most of us are probably distracted dozens of times; every day we get "emergency" e-mails, phone calls, and texts. We take breaks to browse the Internet. Coworkers walk into our offices for a quick chat or send an amusing instant message. It doesn't matter where you work or what you do, you probably deal with distractions on a daily basis. And these distractions are costly: a 2007 study by Basex estimated that distractions cost US businesses $588 billion per year, and this is likely repeated in organizations around the world. Here is the link: http://bit.ly/2HaGKKQInteruptions

What's more (depending on the complexity of your work or project you are on), regaining your concentration after a distraction can take quite a few minutes. If you are distracted ten times a day, multiply the time lost by ten, and it's easy to see why we sometimes don't get much quality work done in a day. Learning how to minimize distractions can dramatically increase your productivity and effectiveness as well as reduce your stress. Without distractions, you can get into the flow, produce high-quality work, and achieve much more each day. This is what keeps your mind free and uncluttered. Here are some examples.

E-mail

While e-mail is incredibly useful, it's also one of the biggest work distractions we face. Many of us could spend entire days simply reading and responding to e-mails. Here are some excellent tips to use to manage this demand:

- **Schedule e-mail times:** Minimize this distraction by scheduling specific times to check and respond to e-mails. For example, you could check e-mail when you first arrive at work, at lunch, and before you leave, and specify a half-hour slot every day to respond to your e-mails. If you do this, it may be useful to let coworkers, customers, and friends know that they will need to contact you another way if it is urgent.
- **Check and respond to e-mail at "low-productivity" times:** Remember that there are certain times of day when you probably do your best work and are most efficient with your time. Some people work best in the morning and others late at night. Schedule your e-mail check-in during your less-productive times, and save your peak hours for doing creative, high-value work.
- **Turn e-mails into actions:** If an e-mail will take more than a few minutes to act on or respond to, add it to your to-do list.
- **Keep your e-mail program closed:** When you're not using your e-mail program, close it entirely, or at least turn off the visual or audible alerts that distract you. This eliminates the temptation to check it constantly.

Disorganization

When your work space or work life is disorganized, it can be difficult to think and plan clearly. A disorganized desk or office can be very distracting. I know this personally for a fact. For years, my office was a complete mess. I wouldn't let my closest of friends or parents, let alone patients, ever see my office. When I had paperwork to do, I would either clear a space or work on top of the paper that was already there.

Well, I finally had enough. I started to work on it, instead of in it. Let me tell you, this was not a fun project. But I knew that I would be happier with a cleaner, more organized office. This took time. A lot of time. I had articles to read, magazines to go through, and files to organize. Once my office started looking cleaner, I started in on drawers and files in old file cabinets. Honestly, I didn't think it would ever end. I kept at it, though, and finally got through it. Is my private office currently perfect? Oh, no. But it is presentable and essentially organized. My recommendation: get your office, desk, and files organized as soon as possible. You will thank yourself for it.

Texting

OMG, I wonder if there is research on how much time is spent texting? Not just how many texts, but how much actual time is spent texting. We would also need to calculate the amount of time we are distracted following each text to fully calculate this. I would be willing to bet most of us would be a bit shocked and perhaps even reconsider how important this activity really is, especially while we are at work. I have experimented with keeping the alert system for texts off to keep this distraction to a minimum. Unless I am expecting something important, I am training myself to answer numerous texts all at the same time. In other words, if you wait for many texts to come through and you answer them all one after another, that would be much more efficient with your time. This adds time and productivity to each day. Training yourself to not look at your phone often is a hard habit to break.

Phone Calls

The ring of the phone has become almost like experiment conducted by Pavlov in 1902 resulting in what is termed "classical conditioning." Here is the link and an old-school video: http://bit.ly/2BqedkbPavlovsDogs. It is worth watching and very interesting in my opinion.

For some reason, we seem to believe that just because someone is calling us that we must answer the call, even if we are working or concentrating and focused on something important. For me, if I don't have time to chat when the call is coming in, I won't answer it, period. Then I will call people back one after another to keep my time efficient.

Minimize phone call distractions by turning your ringer off during your peak work hours. Or let your team know that you won't take nonessential calls between specific times, such as from noon to 2:00 p.m. For me personally, the ringer stays off when I go to bed, every night. Whatever "emergency" comes up, I can deal with beginning at 6:30–7:00 a.m. More recently, while working on this book, the ringer stayed off. If you want to stay focused and keep your mind free from clutter, this is an easy way to minimize distractions.

The Internet

Browsing the web can take up enormous amounts of time from our day, and when we start looking on the Internet for one thing, it frequently leads to something else that we find absolutely fascinating, and this leads to spending another twenty minutes and even two hours before we realize it!

People

Yes, even well-intentioned coworkers and friends can often create distractions. People are all different and frequently waste their own time—and that can mean wasting yours too. Here are some tips to keep in mind for minimizing distractions from other people:

- **Close your door:** Close your office door to keep people from casually stopping by. If they knock or come in anyway, simply explain that when your door is closed, you are working on something important and prefer not to be disturbed unless there's an emergency. Consider working from home or in a conference room when you are working on an important project and don't want to be disturbed.

- **Use headphones:** If you're in a cubicle or open office environment, people are less likely to interrupt you if you're wearing headphones. You can listen to music, a podcast, or your favorite author.
- **Talk to the disrupter:** If you share an office with someone who often disrupts your day, talk to that person about it; the person may not realize he or she is distracting you.

By decreasing your distractions, you actually will have more time to get your work done and your personal errands too. Bottom line, when you get your stuff done, you can relax and have more fun. Is that simple enough?

The Age of Information

It is said that "we live in curious times," and that references not only the Age of Information, but also the Age of Distraction. While we have never been completely free of distractions, from swatting bothersome gnats, flies, or even ants around the outdoor picnic to sorting through piles of incoming mail. Never have the distractions been so voluminous, so overwhelming, so intense, so persistent, as they are now. We have entered this new age of living without being fully aware that it has been happening and without realizing its consequences. Sure, we knew that the Internet and technology were growing, and we were excited about that. It is so easy to search for things - anything. We knew that mobile devices were becoming more and more popular. I mean, who doesn't have a smartphone, right? But, with all that this accessibility to information and staying connected offers us, is it really all a good thing? The constant distractions, the increasing urgency for our attention, the stress that is now associated with constant and relentless multitasking can be, simply put, overwhelming. This feeling of being overwhelmed is not healthy for us, and it could even be considered a social epidemic!

Is It Just Another Addiction?

There is such instant positive feedback to such constant activities as checking e-mail, surfing the web, and checking social networks such as blogs, forums, and Facebook. That's why it's so easy to become addicted to being connected and distracted. Other addictive activities, such as doing drugs or eating junk food, have the same kind of instant positive feedback. You do the activity and right away you're rewarded with something pleasurable, but you don't feel the negative consequences until much later. You check your e-mail and, hey, a new e-mail from a friend! You get a positive feeling, perhaps even a validation of your own self-worth. It feels good to get a message from someone, knowing that person is thinking of you. And this pattern of instant positive feedback rewards you, resulting in checking e-mail more and more frequently until this pattern is solidly ingrained in your daily actions.

Now, years later, you begin to get tired of answering all your e-mail because it has become overwhelming. You may have more important priorities and responsibilities. But usually by then, this pattern you created of constantly checking in is not easy to stop. I have been guilty of this myself. It is ridiculous. How often do we see people that are out and about, and they aren't even talking to one another, but are instead connected to others with their smartphones? I will admit I have been guilty of this too! I understand that we want to stay on top of our newsfeed and read and respond to e-mail and texts, but what about the person who is right there in front of you?

This New Lifestyle

I love this quote by Marcus Aurelius: "Most of what we say and do is not essential. If you can eliminate it, you'll have more time, and more tranquility. Ask yourself at every moment, 'Is this necessary?'" We should probably ask ourselves this question a dozen times each day! I feel that living in the moment, with people, that is what it means to be truly connected.

Being connected by getting constant updates that are just constant distractions has become a part of our lives. Computers have literally taken over our lives. And while I'm as pro technology as the next guy, I also think we need to consider the consequences of this new lifestyle and how it affects our minds.

For me to keep some sanity in this world, I typically separate my day into chunks of time. I will see patients for about three hours, then switch to paperwork for the next few hours. Then I take a break, run errands, exercise, take a nap, and of course fuel my body. I usually only spend time on the phone when I'm out running errands. When it is time to work, I stay focused on that. If I'm on a house project or exercising, I'm focused on that. The more I think about this subject matter as I write about it, I believe focus is a lot like a muscle. You either use it and make it stronger and stronger so it can be of benefit to you, or you will eventually lose it by being distracted throughout your day. We all have the same exact twenty-four hours each and every day. It's always been amazing to me how some "high-performing" people can get so much more done than others with their lives. I believe our focus has a lot to do with that. Here is an excellent resource link: http://bit.ly/2nUvwlSFocus

Living in the Moment

Enjoying life and living in the moment - do you think it is still possible? Well, I do. Am I optimistic? You bet I am. I strive to live right there in the moment by creating memorable events so that I can remember them when I get really, really old, and more importantly, for my mind to be free and at peace. I think of living in the moment with the acronym PTC: Present. Time. Consciousness.

Here are six steps to living in the moment: http://bit.ly/2EDr7NOLivinginTheMoment

1. **Stop thinking about what other people think about you:** To live in the moment and have peace in your mind, focus less on yourself and more on what is going on around you and who you are with. This creates a deeper relationship with friends, loved ones, and even acquaintances.
2. **Worrying is a waste of your time:** Worrying is personally choosing not to be present in the moment. When you trap yourself into thoughts of the past or the future it is impossible to fully participate in the moment in front of you: the right here and the right now. How can that possibly be beneficial to you or your relationships?
3. **Your significant other deserves your attention:** If you have chosen your mate, yet when together, you choose to dwell on other things in the past, present, or future, you are certainly not living in the moment. I believe this will slowly eat away at any relationship given enough time. I have certainly been guilty of this in the past, and I have personally experienced it from the other end as well. Focusing on the present allows your mind to be able to respond thoughtfully, rather than on autopilot. I think we all know how reacting or responding on autopilot works out for us. Usually not good.

4. **Your awareness of time:** We tend to be complete slaves to time. To live in the moment, you must relax and learn what psychologists call "flow." When you are able to relax and focus your mind on what is going on right in front of you, you can reach this state of flow. This is when you lose track of time, your distractions are gone, and your attention and your depth of engagement are at an all-time high. I highly recommend this!
5. **Accept your feelings:** If something is bothering you - some negative thoughts or feelings that you know will resurface and cause a problem - burying them deep down is not going to help. The solution is acceptance by allowing the emotion to be present and feeling it without trying to manipulate, change it, or judge it. Trying to change it or push it away leads to frustration, and that gets exhausting. This is not always easy to do.
6. **Here and now:** We have all had the experience of doing something or driving somewhere only to suddenly realize you forgot what you are doing or missed your exit! Research by Dr. Ellen Langer of Harvard University says this experience is called "mindlessness." This is how you allow life to pass you by. She suggests developing the habit of always noticing something new in whatever situation you are in. This process creates a focus and engagement with the present, allowing you to live in the moment.

Do We Really Need to be Constantly Connected?

"Without great solitude, no serious work is possible."
PABLO PICASSO

While writing this book, I came across this quote. I printed it out and I taped it up next to my monitor as a reminder that this is what it would take to write this book. You see, being constantly connected and distracted comes with a price. The lack of focus can and will affect our peace of mind, our stress levels, and our happiness. In the days when computers took up only part of our lives, there were times when we could get away from it all when we were disconnected from the grid. Unfortunately, many people still filled much of that time with watching television, which isn't necessarily any better. I feel it's important to get away from this constant connectivity; we need some quiet, some time to reflect, some time to contemplate, and some time for solitude. Without it, our minds are constantly bombarded by information and sensations, unable to rest or relax. This results in a constant stress on our minds and bodies in ways that we are not meant to handle.

We need rest. It is important in ways we don't often think about. We need to unplug, and we need to recharge our mental batteries. Quiet, solitude, and reflection lead to greater happiness when they are a part of our daily lives at least to some degree. What you do during this time - read, write, run, nap, sit, watch, listen, have an actual conversation, play, study, build - isn't as important as the simple fact of having that time.

Ideally, I believe this time is best spent with family and friends. Time spent cultivating healthy relationships with others is the best way to spend your time.

In the following chapter, we learn more about the importance of the food we eat that fuels our body. There is a lot to learn there, enjoy!

Fuel for Your Body

This chapter on fueling your body is not meant to be an actual nutrition or diet book, but far more than that. It is meant to give you a deeper understanding how your body functions and also give you some insider secrets to help you make smart and healthy choices for you and your family. With the information and education, you receive from this chapter, especially if you follow the links I have given to you, you will amass a wealth of knowledge regarding nutrition and healthy living.

For Quality Food, Think Organic

First off, organic foods are a must! I was born and raised in the Central Valley of California in the city of Fresno. We were used to lots of fresh fruits and vegetables. In my family's own back yard, we grew pomegranates, apricots, strawberries, and tomatoes! On the outskirts of town, there were orchards full of fruits, vegetables, nuts, and dairy farms. Supposedly, the Central Valley had some of the most fertile soil for planting and growing produce. When I was young, I didn't even think about or concern myself with the pesticides being sprayed on these foods. When you are raised in this type of environment, you simply assume everything is healthy for you. I highly recommend the documentary on Netflix, called *Food, Inc.* You can watch the documentary for free at this YouTube link: http://imdb.to/1WTpcas It will open your eyes to how your food is processed, and believe me, it is a shocker! I recommend for everyone to do a little research on your own so that you become knowledgeable about the food you eat. I realize that organic foods are more expensive; however, if you factor in the cost of poor health and the resulting medical costs that will be necessary, you will soon realize it is in your best interest in developing the healthy bodies that we all need.

Genetically Modified Organisms

GMOs were first introduced into grocery stores in 1994 as the "Flavr Savr," tomato. It was genetically made so that it would take much longer to spoil and keep its firmness longer. By 1999, over 100 million acres worldwide were being planted and farmed with GMO seeds. By 2003, GMO-resistant insects had appeared with a brand-new bacterium called Bt toxin. By 2011, these toxins were now being found in the blood supply of pregnant women, showing evidence it is being passed to fetuses. In 2015, there were billions of GMO acres being farmed. The supposed master plan is that the GMO seeds and plants are better to tolerate the chemicals being sprayed on them, "genetically." The manufacturer of the GMO seeds just so happens to be the *same manufacturer* of the chemicals that are being sprayed on those plants. It has been well documented that foods grown from GMOs are dangerous and not considered healthy for your body. If you are not familiar with GMO products by now, you need to start studying ASAP! Here is a link from Dr. Mercola that I recommend: http://bit.ly/2smuS5cDangerGMO The biggest manufacturer of GMO in the United States is the company Monsanto. According to Bloomberg, Monsanto is the third-most-hated company in America http://bloom.bg/1TO1V9I This company is more than huge; it is extremely profitable, specializes in chemicals, and is most noted for its GMO seeds, pesticide chemicals, for being a corporate bully, and for suing other farmers. Over 90 percent of the corn and soybeans produced in the United States are now genetically modified and used for animal feed and ethanol fuel. These crops are also used for the corn syrup, found in sweetened beverages and soy lecithin in chocolate bars. Monsanto's weed-killer product that they designed for their own GMO seeds is called Roundup. Their gross revenues in 2015 for this product alone was $4.76 billion. Monsanto is dominating and monopolizing our country's farmlands.

Let me take you back a few dozen years to the Vietnam War. In the 1960s, Monsanto was the company that made the chemical that was used in Vietnam to kill the foliage so the troops could move through the jungles; it was called "Agent Orange." Unfortunately, when they sprayed this chemical in the jungle they also sprayed it directly on our troops. The damage this chemical has done to our veterans is long lasting and has caused irreparable human suffering. Here is a link for more information on this: http://1.usa.gov/1OlIZHD. Agent Orange is directly linked to amyloidosis, chronic Leukemia, chloracne, type 2 diabetes, Hodgkin's lymphoma, ischemic heart disease, multiple myeloma, Parkinson's Disease, peripheral neuropathy, porphyria cutanea tarda, prostate cancer, respiratory cancers (lung), and soft-tissue sarcoma. Roundup is said to be the Agent Orange of our time.

Processed Foods

It really is just this simple: **stay away from processed foods**. But, you might ask, what exactly is a processed food? Isn't every food to some degree a processed food? Well, yes, of course, it must be processed to some degree before you can buy it at the store. If you are fortunate enough to grow your own food, you know exactly what it takes to plant, grow, harvest, and bring it directly to your table for your family. While this is a process, it's the healthiest food for your body if you garden without pesticides and herbicides.

In general, when you buy a product from the grocery store in a box or a can, it has typically been processed in a manner that will not benefit you becoming healthier. What about fast food, you ask? Do you think that has been processed very much? Fast food is simply poison for your body! It has added sugar, tons of salt, and the meat that is used is simply no good! Check out the documentary on Netflix called *Super Size Me*; I highly recommend it. Morgan Spurlock purposefully ate at McDonalds for thirty days in a row. Breakfast, lunch, and dinner. He documents his journey and utilizes not one, but three doctors to monitor his health. Here is a free YouTube link if you don't have Netflix: http://bit.ly/2o3sYkvSuperSizeMe

Wait, what about the salads? They must be healthy for you, right? They are not if they come from a fast-food restaurant! They will be typically laced with added sugar, salt, and for crying out loud, please don't eat those disgusting croutons!

What are Superfoods?

WebMD states that superfoods are antioxidant-rich fruits, vegetables, and herbs to include in your daily diet that help to strengthen your immune system and your ability to fight infection and disease. Here is the list I recommend:

Protein and Amino Acids: Amaranth, camu-camu, goji berry, sacha inchi, sprouted quinoa, whey protein. These help the body build lean muscle, heal wounds, and improve skin and hair. They support optimal brain function, mental clarity, improved mood, and reduced cravings.

Antioxidants—Red Superfoods: Açai berry, Acerola cherry, bilberry, camu-camu, goji berry, grape-seed extract, green tea, maca root, pomegranate. These helps to reduce oxidative damage in the body caused by free radicals. Oxidative damage is a major cause for degenerative (aging) conditions such as heart disease, high blood pressure, dementia, and arthritis.

Phytonutrients—Green Superfoods: Barley grass, blue-green algae, chia seeds, chlorella, flax, grape-seed extract, hydrilla, spinach, spirulina, sprouted quinoa, wheat grass. These boost immunity, helps fight disease, help to slow down the aging process, detoxify the body, and have alkalizing properties.

Adaptogens: Ashwagandha, astragalus, cordyceps, holy basil leaf, maca root, reishi mushroom, schisandra, suma root. These plant-derived agents help to adapt the body and to protect it from stress. Adaptogenic herbs are unique from other substances in their ability to balance endocrine hormones and the immune system.

Prebiotics: Pea fiber, yacon root. These promote better intestinal health and stimulate growth of friendly bacteria for better digestion.

Digestive Enzymes: Amylase, bromelain from pineapple, cellulose, lactase, lipase, papain from papaya, protease. These help the body break down foods and increase absorption of nutrients.

How Often Should You Eat?

Most current philosophies agree that skipping breakfast is a bad idea. You want some "fuel" for your body for energy, and that is what food is: it is simply fuel for your body. If you want your body to be healthy, you feed it with premium fuel, period. One popular philosophy that I believe in is eating smaller and very regular meals. These meals must be portion controlled with the correct amount of nutrition. I recommend this link for you to learn more about portions: http://bit.ly/2H6zDDrSmallMeals. We have a portion-control system in our office that is part of our weight-loss programs.

The plan is to stay within your calorie goals, but the premise is to eat smaller meals frequently. I also recommend mixing things up a bit sort of like confusing your body to keep it guessing. I personally do some modified intermittent fasting from time to time. This is a little more of an advanced technique, however. Here is a link to learn more about it: http://bit.ly/2EzPrQvIntermittentFasting

I personally do a combination of the two. One or maybe two days per week, I won't eat much for dinner and then try to put off eating in the morning for as long as I can. I always drink plenty of water during this time, as it is important to continue to hydrate. We have programs available that can be custom-tailored to you and a coaching program to help you through them to reach your goals.

How Your Body Assimilates Food

As we get older, our bodies do not assimilate or absorb foods at the same level of efficiency as when we were younger. Now, you can jump up and down about this and get upset with this statement. However, these are the facts, and they will not change. As most of us know by now, we can get away with a lot of mischief when we are younger, but getting older, well, let's just say it "isn't for sissies." You must make significant changes, especially in the way that you nourish and feed your body.

The lining of our intestines is where the body absorbs all of the nutrition from what we consume, and that is where the digestion process begins in our body. As we mature, however, our intestinal lining loses some of its ability to absorb nutrients from our food. Therefore, we lose our ability to assimilate vital proteins, carbs, vitamins, nutrients, and minerals as efficiently as when we were younger. Therefore, we must continue to practice better and cleaner nutrition for our bodies if our goal is to stay healthy or become healthier. You can learn more about this at this link: http://wb.md/1x0Rljj

When consulting with patients about nutrition and eating properly, I had a patient that informed me that "not everybody's body is the same." Meaning, not all nutrition or diet plans will work for everybody. She has struggled with her weight most of her life. I couldn't agree with her more. Additionally, we all don't have the same biochemistry, genetics, schedules, work environments, responsibilities, sleep patterns, willingness to consistently exercise, or the same commitment to a proven system. The list goes on and on, and in fact, I have never met two people who are exactly the same. I've even noticed differences in people who are twins!

Clean Eating and Meal Preparation

The basics of clean eating and healthy living are the foundation for getting your body healthier and sexier, having more energy, improving your self-image, and getting off and staying off dangerous drugs and medications.

Meal preparation has been found to be a very successful way to plan your portion control, and it is especially important when you are on a busy schedule. Personally, I eat almost all of my meals at home, and I come home for lunch too. Not many busy people have that opportunity, so meal prepping is a foundation principle that I highly recommend. You can meal prep in the morning before you leave for the day or do your prepping the night before. However, the most successful meal preppers prepare on Sunday for their week!

Does this take planning? You bet it does. Listen, if this were easy, everyone would be healthy, no one would be overweight, and there would be no chronic or metabolic diseases. We would have minimal heart disease, cancer, diabetes, or obesity.

By now, we all know the facts: we have real issues with our health in this country. The website Newser.com published in 2015 that the United States is rated a pathetic number thirty-three on the list of the healthiest countries in the world. Here's a link to the healthiest countries in case you are thinking of moving: http://bit.ly/2ssH1WgTopHealthyCountries

Getting healthy, being healthy, and staying healthy takes work! Meal prepping is a big part of that work. When you plan your meals for the week, it takes all the thinking out of what you are going to eat in that moment. You know, that moment of, "OMG, I'm starving right now, and I must eat something—anything." We've all been there, and we all know how that works out, don't we?

The basics, however, will always be the basics. And this is where we need to begin. Some people—and dare I say, most people—are literally led around by their mouths. They may label themselves as "foodies," and therefore must always have food that is tasty. Well, tasty usually means it will have plenty of unhealthy additives such as fat and sugar to make it taste that way.

I try not to eat out very often. The reason for this is very simple. It just tastes too damn good. In my opinion, you need to train your mouth. Yes, I said it: train your mouth! When the food you eat is super tasty, it becomes irresistible, and what do you think happens? We want more of it, don't we? Which leads to overeating.

Overeating

I remember a TV commercial many years ago with the tagline, "I can't believe I ate the whole thing." This was a very successful ad campaign from 1972 for the product, Alka-Seltzer. The basic selling premise was, you already *know* that you are going to overeat, so when you do, just take Alka-Seltzer and all will be well. This ad campaign was huge for the company and on a subliminal level made it OK to overeat because there was immediate help for you and your poor upset stomach. Here is the YouTube link for that ad from back in the day: http://bit.ly/2BrVcxWICantBelieve

I remember a family from the office many years ago who I still stay in touch with through the magic of Facebook. The mom, Janet, came into the office for treatment and mentioned she was concerned that her son had been sick the day before. He had vomited, and she was wondering if she should take him to the pediatrician or even to the hospital emergency room. I asked her some questions about where her son had been and what had been eating earlier that day or perhaps the day before that. She described a lavish birthday party he had attended and how much fun he had. There was so much food for everyone—even the parents too. I asked if her son had eaten much that day. She immediately commented, "Oh, yes," and expressed concerned that maybe he had food poisoning. I asked her what he had eaten, and she explained that, over the course of the afternoon, he had eaten a hamburger, a hotdog, chips, cookies, and cake and ice cream too. Of course, this was all washed down with Coke or soda of some kind. Being familiar with her son, I asked if he had been running around much during the party. Her response was immediate: "Oh, absolutely, there was even a bouncy house for all the kids," she said proudly. Sounds like a great party!

So, let's just imagine for a moment if we were that little boy's tummy. You consume all that "food" and mix in the junk food too. Stir it all up in this small little belly, then jump up and down for a few hours, then run around in circles like most kids do when they are high on sugar, and what do you think will happen? Yep, he threw it up! That sounds like pretty normal physiology to me. If I was that little tummy, I would want to get rid of all that too. I suggested that his mom give him a day and see how he was feeling. Sure enough, the next day he was fine. No doctor's visit, no emergency-room visit, no x-rays, no CT scans, no MRIs, no shots, no pills. Nada.

In some circles and certainly in some families it is a badge of honor if we can eat a lot of food. There is absolutely nothing about this that is healthy for you. Please check out the documentary on Netflix called *Fed Up*. It is on childhood obesity, and it is a must watch. Here is a Netflix link I found: http://nflx.it/1sW4NFK. Please be mindful of the amount of food and especially junk food that you put into your mouth and your children's mouths. Train your mouth to eat less and train it to eat foods that are healthy and are not full of sugar, salt, and fat. Is this necessarily easy to do? Of course not. It takes work, and it certainly takes discipline!

Cleansing and the Dreaded Detox

We know we need to do it. Yet we are all a little panicky about it and not really sure what to actually do. If you have done it before or you do it on a regular basis, then you know it really is no big deal. Bottom line, we should all do an occasional intestinal cleanse! Let's look at this realistically.

Spring Cleaning Any Time of the Year

You clean your home, your car, your hair, your body. Literally everything gets cleaned. So, why *not* your intestines? I think the biggest concern for people is how their body will react to the cleanse. When consulting with patients about this, the first question is, "Will I be able to leave the house, or will I have to live in my bathroom?" I do understand this concern. I've lived in the bathroom before and it is no party. But most people don't have time for that. For me, I think the smart move is a gentle cleansing on a semiregular basis. You have to remove and eliminate the toxins from your system, period. We have products and systems in place to offer our patients that are very simple. For me, simplicity will always be the key. You may contact our office, visit our website, or do some searching on your own.

The Body's Natural Detox System

Oftentimes, people don't realize that the body has its own extraordinary internal detoxification system. Here's a brief look at three critical organs involved:

- **The Liver:** Your first line of defense against toxins that are digested is your liver, which acts like a filter in preventing toxic substances contained in foods from passing into your bloodstream.
- **The Colon:** This organ has bacteria that produce both healthy and unhealthy chemicals. You want to keep your colon flowing regularly since its main role is to flush out toxic chemicals before they can do you any harm.
- **The Kidneys:** Like clockwork, the kidneys are constantly filtering your blood and getting rid of toxins in the form of urine.

Foods that are known to benefit these organs:

The Liver: Dark berries such as blueberries and blackberries will make it easier for your liver to get rid of certain toxins. Hot peppers have capsaicin, which boosts enzymes responsible for detoxifying the liver. As a rule, the hotter the pepper, the more capsaicin.

The Colon: Whole grains contain phosphorous, a natural laxative, and fiber to help bulk up your stools. Fermented foods like kimchi (Korean spicy pickled cabbage) and sour pickles are packed with probiotics, the good bacteria that help protect your colon.

The Kidneys: Soy products such as miso, tofu, and edamame all act like diuretics, allowing you to urinate more often. (Personally, I'm not a fan of anything soy based). Cruciferous vegetables such as cauliflower, bok choy, and broccoli increase your kidneys' ability to transport toxins into the urine and help liver cells recover from detox.

Twelve Detox Foods You May Already Have in Your Kitchen:

Ginger: Ginger helps to start the day off right and is easy to add to a variety of drinks, smoothies, and foods. Ginger can help to settle your stomach and contains a number of antioxidants that can help neutralize harmful compounds made by your body.

Beets: Slice them and use them to add color to your plate or put in salad. Beets are rich in a variety of vitamins and minerals. They also contain a variety of phytochemicals that are good for your body. As a bonus, beets are sweet but also high in fiber, so they won't spike your blood sugar.

Garlic: Garlic has long been known for its health benefits. It contains several vitamins and a variety of minerals in a surprisingly small package. The key to garlic is you need to eat it raw. Crushing it before use helps release the compound allicin, which has a variety of positive health benefits.

Artichokes: Artichokes are high in fiber and contain a significant amount of vitamin C, potassium, and magnesium. The leaves contain a compound that helps with bile release and aids digestion.

Green Tea: Packed with phytochemicals and antioxidants, green tea can help your body recover from detoxifying the blood and from the daily wear and tear of generating energy. Add some ginger for a truly rejuvenating warm drink.

Apples: If you're seeking some sweetness, grab an apple. Packed with fiber and spanning the spectrum of vitamins and minerals, apples are an easily transportable way to get your body the nutrients it needs every day. Plus, biting into an apple can help to clean your teeth naturally.

Broccoli: Few people know that broccoli contains huge amounts of vitamin C. One cup has 135 percent of the amount needed daily. In addition, it's loaded with B vitamins, which are essential to a variety of the body's daily functions. Broccoli is also high in vitamin K, which is important for your liver's production of clotting factors for the blood.

Cinnamon: Common in every American kitchen, cinnamon is a great way to boost the flavor of a meal or smoothie. Cinnamon has some antibacterial activity and is rich in antioxidants.

Parsley: While often discarded as a meal garnish, parsley is dense in a variety of vitamins and minerals, particularly vitamins C, E, and K. It also contains iron. Throw it in as seasoning on a variety of dishes or make it a key ingredient of your next soup.

Olive Oil: A healthy favorite that can be drizzled on any number of foods, olive oil is high in healthy mono- and polyunsaturated fats. It also contains vitamins E and K.

Almonds: Looking for a healthy snack that will keep you feeling full during a cleanse? Try almonds. These nuts are high in protein, which keeps you feeling full longer. They're also loaded with calcium, magnesium, and plenty of fiber.

Basil: Basil contains large amounts of flavonoids that can help to soak up free radicals and stave off cancer. It may also help to reduce inflammation by blocking the same chemical pathways as aspirin and acetaminophen. It makes a great flavor addition to any dish.

I have personally been cleansing for over twenty years. I don't necessarily do it every week or even every month, but sometimes I do. I routinely take personal inventory on what I've been eating, my levels of stress, and the hours I work to determine if it is time to cleanse or not. I don't want to cleanse too often, as this doesn't allow the body to perform its normal physiological functions on its own.

For more information you may call our office, visit our website or you may schedule a private on-line consultation at https://calendly.com/drkoehlerconsult to discuss your specific needs. We look forward to helping you on your journey to improving your health.

The next chapter on mobility and increasing your energy may give you just the right motivation to get started and stay on track!

Mobility and Increasing Your Energy

In our world, everything we see and do is based on energy. Without energy, it is over. No electricity, no lights, no cars, no food, no water. The human body, though, is very interesting when it comes to energy. The way it works is that **our bodies produce energy from the food we eat.** Our bodies break down the food in our digestive system, and the food mixes with fluids (acids and enzymes) in the stomach. This results in glucose, which is like the gasoline or fuel we put into our car. When this glucose is absorbed and released into the bloodstream, it can be used immediately for energy, or it can be stored in the body to potentially be used later. This stored energy eventually turns to fat! Let's sum this up: **the food we eat turns into fuel and gives our bodies energy.** Next, we will attempt to apply some good ol' fashioned common sense.

If we were to supply our body with—wait for it—junk food, it will result in poor energy and poor performance. I know, I know, this is a tough concept for some of us to grasp. So, let's try this again. This time let's use one of those analogy things.

So, let's say you saved up and finally bought yourself the car of your dreams, and you actually got the model with that really good engine. It doesn't matter if it's the high-performance engine (my fav), or the super-efficient fuel-economy engine. Both engines are designed specifically for different purposes, and they will only run their best when given the exact fuel they are designed for. Now, if you decide that you just don't care about what your engine needs to perform at its best, that's of course up to you. You are the decision-maker. If you give your car that cheap watered-down version of fuel or one with a boatload of added sugar, fat, and chemicals, how do you think your car will perform?

Stay with me on this. When your car was new, it had a lot of pep, and it might not have even missed a beat in the beginning. But when your car gets a little older, shall we say, with few more miles on the odometer, it starts really losing some of that pep. It loses its efficiency, and the performance begins to decline. You could say that it just doesn't have that same "get-up-and-go" that it used to. What makes it even worse is that now it starts breaking down on you.

No big surprise then, right? Our bodies use food for energy, and when you give your body food without nutritional value (junk food), your body loses its energy and performance and eventually starts to break down on you. And when you don't burn off that extra fuel (calories), it goes right into your storage tank and becomes stored as fat.

OK, so let's reevaluate this for a moment. If we were to put into our bodies the proper fuel (food) and proper amount of fuel, that would be a pretty good combination, right? And for any extra fuel we put in, we will need to burn that off. So how are we going to do that? I know, you already know the answer, don't you? Yep, it's exercise. Oh snap, you didn't want me to use that dreaded word "exercise," did you? Well, sorry, this book is about you and improving your health, and if you want someone to lie to you, you will need go elsewhere! I will make you a deal though. How about instead of calling it exercise, we call it mobility? That's a pretty cool word, isn't it?

Mobility

Let's talk more about this mobility then, shall we? I've got a quick question for you. Do you think that you will need to practice mobility to improve your health, get and stay healthy, get off the medications, lose weight, sleep better, have more energy, have a better sex life, have a better attitude, decrease stress, reduce anxiety, and help with depression on a regular or consistent basis? Do you know the answer yet? Well, you are correct, the answer is yes! I'll bet you knew the answer all along, didn't you? On a quick side note, my research tells me only smart people will even read this book, so you being right about this makes a lot of sense to me.

This mobility of which we speak has been proven, much like exercise, to have a positive impact in about every aspect of your life. It literally is one of the key components in preventing and reversing chronic disease in our bodies.

Since it has been scientifically proven to help you, why in the world wouldn't you want to work on your mobility *daily* if it really is that beneficial? Here are just a few examples of what mobility can do for you and your health according to the CDC: http://1.usa.gov/1JDovX9.

1. Controls your weight
2. Reduces your risk of cardiovascular disease
3. Reduces your risk for type 2 diabetes and metabolic syndrome
4. Reduces your risk of some cancers
5. Strengthens your bones and muscles
6. Improves your mental health and mood
7. Improves your ability to do daily activities and prevent falls when older
8. Increases your chance of living longer

I must say, this really is an impressive list. Who in their right mind wouldn't want to practice their mobility every single day or at least three to four times per week? The bottom line here is, the more mobility you do, the healthier your body will be and the less medication you will need to take. By the way, this is all part of my "master plan" for getting your body, mind, and attitude right and taking your health to the next level!

You Will Need a System

So, what are we going to do about this whole topic of mobility when the statistics say that **you really don't want to do it**. Obviously, you will need to start with something simple. I typically suggest starting with some type of mobility that you will be willing to do on a regular basis. Yes, I do mean consistently. In fact, consistency will always be the key to your success with mobility. Some people love to exercise and are willing to practice their mobility all day long. For the rest of us, well, not so much. But when you have an actual system in place, it takes all the thinking and guesswork out of it. It creates a routine for your mobility. Doesn't that sound exciting? Yeah, I know, not so much. But remember you don't have to do it.

The truth is, by simply eating correctly, you can and will get healthier, and you will certainly lose weight simply by eating better. So, we could just stop right here, couldn't we? Are you starting to understand and learn a little bit about me?

I know and understand the benefits of this mobility, and I have applied them to my own life and have gotten amazing results even well into my fifties, so I'm not ready to give up on you either!

Listen, I personally don't plan on trying to keep up with everyone, and you don't have to either. I have patients and friends who have received their black belts in martial arts, who are professional baseball players, high-end competitive surfers, semiprofessional volleyball players, marathon runners, and competitors in Ironman races and body-building competitions. I have treated dozens of collegiate athletes and some professional athletes too. For me, I simply stay consistent with the system that I have found works best for me, my schedule, and my fitness goals.

Having a system in place will work for you too. I love helping injured people in pain get well and helping them take their health and their fitness to the next level. Do you want to know why? Because I hate—and I mean, hate—all the drugs and medications that people are taking. Although, I do realize some of them may be absolutely necessary to keep you alive.

One of my best friends needed a kidney transplant a couple of years ago; through bad luck of the draw, and he was dealt a congenital kidney disorder. It is a miracle that he is alive today. His wife donated one of her kidneys to him, and she will always be his true hero for the rest of his life. He must continue to be on medications or he will die.

Most of us are not in that situation and will never need to be either. Most of us, with a little bit of direction and a little bit of work, can turn our health around by changing our lifestyle choices and, of course, adding some mobility.

What is the Correct Amount of Mobility?

The correct amount of mobility for you is very dependent on where you are currently at with your body and your schedule. For some of you, a light stretching program would be a great start. It could be a daily walk, bicycle ride, swimming, or going to the gym. Whatever it is, you need to start and have a system in place that will work with your schedule.

Here is a quick example. There is a big difference in what type of exercise you can and should be doing if you are ten pounds overweight versus one hundred pounds overweight. Look, we don't have time for injuries here because more than likely we are already dealing with some injuries that are already slowing us down. So we must be smart about this and start with a very reasonable amount of mobility in the beginning. It's the smart thing and the right thing to do.

We are currently working on a video series of short exercise routines. Come on, who can't a few minutes to exercise, right? For others, a more advanced program can be recommended that is based on HIIT, or high-intensity interval training. Believe me, eventually this is where you want to be. This type of program is designed to kick you in the behind and give you some amazing results.

When you are getting "back into it," I always recommend patients to go slow in the beginning. Because as soon as you are injured in the process, everything comes to a screeching halt, stopping your momentum, and that doesn't boost morale or improve motivation. Furthermore, it will take time to heal, and you may now need treatment or rehab before you can get back on track. It is always smarter to start a bit slower and build up to the serious HIIT programs like P90X, Turbofire, bootcamps, CrossFit, gyms, and personal trainers.

Personally, I've had a gym membership for thirty years, and I do go on occasion, but I prefer to work out in my home gym with my system. Back in the day, I spent plenty of time in the gym and truthfully it was as much social as it was for exercise. Today, it's different; when I exercise, I'm very focused so I can get it done, get the results I'm looking for, and move on to the next thing. Personally, I don't love exercise—oops, I meant mobility. What I do love is the effect that it has on my body and mind.

You will need to take personal inventory on the type of mobility you are willing to participate in. There are so many types it is endless. We don't always get to do our favorite mobility every day, so my suggestion is to be flexible about it, have a system in place, and most importantly, be consistent.

Building Muscle

Now I would like to talk about building muscle. Almost no matter the situation, your health or medical condition, how much you weigh, or how much you need to lose, building muscle is very important. Building muscle actually speeds up your metabolism so that your body will burn more fat naturally. The latest research on type 2 diabetes? Yep, eat right and build more muscle! With the right plan and the right system in place, it really is possible to get off the medications. Here are two links on diabetes, exercise, and weight training that will provide you with some excellent research. I recommend you read them both: http://bit.ly/1YxM0u0DiabetesExercise, http://wb.md/1WCb7Ow.

To build more muscle, you must eat correctly, typically ingesting more protein. I personally only eat lean protein from animals, fish, eggs, beans, and legumes that are organic. I frequently use protein and superfood shakes almost daily. For the ladies, please don't tell me about your fears of looking like a man with a lot of muscles or looking like a bodybuilder—it's just not going to happen. The word is "testosterone" and you will never make enough of it. For us guys, each year we unfortunately will naturally lose some of our testosterone production, so eating right and building muscle is the key to keeping our youth and increasing energy.

If you want to schedule a consultation with me regarding the best exercise and nutritional plan for you, call our office and we can make an appointment for you.

The next chapter is on sleep. I am a super-fan of getting enough rest!

Sleep: Recharging Your Battery

Sleep is a funny thing, isn't it? I remember as a kid that I never wanted to go to bed. I would sneak out of bed and peek around the wall into the living room where my parents were watching TV. "Go to bed," were the dreaded words I never wanted to hear, and this was the beginning of my understanding that my parents really did have eyes in the backs of their heads as they never even turned around! Do you remember your parents telling you that you look tired, that you needed to "get some rest," and that you were going to bed, "*right now*!"? That was the worst ever because I knew there was no negotiation at that point. As parents, you can take one look at your children and can tell that they need to get more rest.

As adults, we seem to know much better than anybody else about ourselves, and we certainly don't want to be told what to do. If you tell people they look tired, it seems this is considered an insult and has become socially inappropriate and even considered a rude thing to say. Can you imagine this: "Geez Mary, you don't look so good today and you look tired"? Even worse, if a man were to say that to a woman. Most of us guys have probably learned the hard way that this will never work out well, even if it is well intentioned.

In my research on sleep, the documentary *Sleepless in America* by *National Geographic* really stands out. I highly recommend spending an hour and a half educating yourself on this subject. Here is the link: http://bit.ly/1UaY9RESleeplessinAmerica. According to the research, "40 percent of American adults are sleep deprived." Here are some additional facts about sleep:

- Americans sleep about two hours less per night than we used to fifty years ago.
- Over half of American adults—65 percent of them—sleep with cell phones next to their beds.
- Too little sleep for one week can turn a healthy person into a prediabetic.
- Large portions of the population—40 percent of American adults and 70 percent of adolescents—are sleep deprived.
- Lack of sleep increases appetite for fatty foods by 33 percent.
- Alcohol interrupts our normal pattern of quality sleep.
- Lack of sleep weakens your body's immune system.
- In the lab, cancer grows twice as fast in animals with disrupted sleep.
- Sleep deprivation impairs memory and learning.
- 70 percent of American high school students fail to get enough sleep per night.
- Lack of sleep is linked to obesity, diabetes, Alzheimer's disease, cancer, and cardiovascular disease.
- Insomnia is associated with depression and anxiety disorders.
- Insomnia is more common in women and increases with age.
- Medications commonly interrupt our normal sleep patterns.
- Sleep medications have the same side effects as not getting enough sleep: drowsiness, dizziness, memory loss, and abnormal thoughts and behavior.
- The most common cause of sleep apnea is being overweight.
- Lack of sleep reduces the overall performance of your mind and body.
- NASA research show that naps improve on-the-job performance of military pilots by 34 percent and alertness by 100 percent.

You Know You Need the Rest

So how much sleep do we really need? It will depend just a bit on the person and what is going on in his or her life. If a person is on medications and has heavy stress, emotional issues, sleep apnea, lots of physical or mental work, physical exercise, overeating, or obesity, these condition result in not sleeping well. Most experts agree the magic number is a minimum of seven hours per night. The Mayo Clinic has a pretty cool guideline on the right amount of sleep based on your age and other factors and is worth checking out: http://mayocl.in/1GBFaZp.

Age group	Recommended amount of sleep
Newborns	14 to 17 hours a day
12 months	About 10 hours at night, plus 4 hours of naps
2 years	About 11 to 12 hours at night, plus a 1- to 2-hour afternoon nap
3 to 5 years	10 to 13 hours
6 to 13 years	9 to 11 hours
14 to 17 years	8 to 10 hours
Adults	7 to 9 hours

In addition to age, other factors affect how many hours of sleep you need. For example:

- **Pregnancy.** Changes in the body during early pregnancy can increase the need for sleep.
- **Aging.** Older adults need about the same amount of sleep as younger adults. As you get older, however, your sleep patterns might change. Older adults tend to sleep more lightly and for a shorter period of time than do younger adults.
- **Previous sleep deprivation.** If you're sleep deprived, the amount of sleep you need increases.
- **Sleep quality.** If your sleep is frequently interrupted, you're not getting quality sleep. The quality of your sleep is just as important as the quantity.

Take a Nap

Some people claim to feel rested on just a few hours of sleep a night, but research tells us their performance is affected. I feel a bit sorry for people who say, "Oh, I can't nap." These are typically the same people who don't sleep well at night either. I was personally taught by a mentor of mine long ago to go home for lunch and take a nap, which I do about five to six days per week on average. To do this, I set my life up to live and work in the same zip code. This has saved hours and hours of time commuting. As I'm writing on this topic right now, I'm starting to think about taking my nap. I absolutely love my naps, and I don't plan on ever giving those up.

As I frequently multitask throughout my day, I may be short on time and only get ten to fifteen minutes to nap. Other times, it may be an hour or more. If possible, I prefer to allow my body to wake up on its own without the use of an alarm clock. That way I know that I am rested. During the week, I always use an alarm clock, though, just in case. Waking up on my own I feel is a more normal way of providing my body the right amount of sleep it needs. Here is an interesting list of famous celebrities who were well known for their napping:

- **Leonardo da Vinci** took multiple naps a day and slept less at night.
- The French emperor **Napoleon** was known for taking naps. It was routine.
- Physicist **Albert Einstein** napped each day, on top of getting ten hours of sleep each night.
- **Thomas Edison** boasted about needing very little sleep. He was a bit embarrassed about his napping habits; he napped daily and stated that he got energy from them.
- **Eleanor Roosevelt** used to boost her energy by napping before speaking engagements.
- **Gene Autry**, the "Singing Cowboy," routinely took naps in his dressing room between performances.
- President **John F. Kennedy** ate his lunch in bed and then settled in for a nap every day.
- **John D. Rockefeller** napped every afternoon in his office.
- **Winston Churchill's** afternoon nap was "nonnegotiable." He believed it helped him get twice as much done each day.
- President **Lyndon B. Johnson** took a nap every afternoon at 3:30 p.m. to break his day up into "two shifts."
- President **Ronald Reagan** was famous for taking his naps.
- President **Bill Clinton** relied heavily on naps while in the White House.
- **Margaret Thatcher** had a set napping schedule between 2:30 p.m. and 3:30 p.m.

- **Arnold Schwarzenegger** stated he appreciates his naps in the afternoon.
- **Salvador Dali** was said to have invented the micronap.
- **Muhammad Ali** would train in the afternoon after his nap.
- **Aristotle** believed in the power of napping for inspiration and genius.
- **Charles Darwin** scheduled his naps between 3:00 p.m. and 4:00 p.m. every day.

You will notice this is big group of *older* people, right? Remember, they weren't old in their day. They were the thought leaders, the movers and shakers of their times. Researching this topic of sleep, it is quite apparent there is a lack of younger, professional and entrepreneurial people admitting to napping. I believe people today either don't understand the importance of proper rest and napping, or it is simply not cool to admit to in this busy society of ours. Regardless, I've been napping since my thirties and have found it very beneficial for health, relaxation, and energy.

Benefits of Napping

Consider taking a daily nap for the following five reasons:

- **A nap restores alertness:** You know how your energy dips in the early afternoon? You start feeling a little sleepy and lose focus. It happens to most of us. A quick nap can bring us right back up to speed. The National Sleep Foundation recommends a short nap of twenty to thirty minutes, "for improved alertness and performance without leaving you feeling groggy or interfering with nighttime sleep." Here is a cool video to check out on napping: http://bit.ly/2nZrk3oSleepEnergy
- **A nap prevents burnout:** In our "always-on" culture, we go, go, go. However, we were not meant to race without rest. Doing so leads to stress, frustration, and burnout. Taking a simple nap is like a system reboot. It relieves stress and gives you a fresh start. Research subjects who nap show greater emotional resilience, improved cognitive function, and much more. Just thirty minutes can prevent the day's wear and tear from frying your circuits.

- **A nap heightens sensory perception:** According to Dr. Sara C. Mednick, author of *Take a Nap, Change Your Life,* napping can restore the sensitivity of sight, hearing, and taste. Napping also improves your creativity by relaxing your mind and allowing new associations to form. When it comes to making new brain connections, nappers had the edge in research.
- **A nap reduces the risk of heart disease:** Did you know those who take a midday siesta at least three times a week are 37 percent less likely to die of heart disease? Working men are 64 percent less likely. In a 2007 study published in the *Archives of Internal Medicine,* Dr. Dimitrios Trichopoulos of the Harvard School of Public Health in Boston, who led the study, said, "Taking a nap could turn out to be an important weapon in the fight against coronary mortality."
- **A nap makes you more productive.** The secret to becoming more productive is not managing your *time,* it's managing your *energy.* Numerous studies have shown workers becoming increasingly unproductive as the day wears on. Just think of your own experience. This link will explain the research at Harvard University: http://bit.ly/2CiNkM0HarvardResearch demonstrates that a thirty-minute nap boosted the performance of workers, returning their productivity to beginning-of-the-day levels.

To create better sleep patterns, you need to establish a regular routine. It appears that going to bed at regular time—and most importantly, waking up at a regular time—helps train your body into a routine of regular sleep. You will also want to make your room as dark and quite as possible. It has also been shown that a room that is on the cool side will improve your night's sleep. Lastly, you want to take as much media and technology out of the bedroom as possible and establish your bedroom as your sanctuary for relaxation and sleep.

The following chapter is on water. The importance of proper water intake can never be overstated. You will also want a filtration system, or you will become the filter!

Water: Your Core Energy Source

Your brain is made up of 75 percent water! Your body is made up of approximately 60 percent water, and your lungs are made up of 83 percent water. That is a lot of water! Water is essential for your body to function. Just think about this for a moment: if our bodies consist of that much water, why don't we pay more attention to making sure that we stay hydrated throughout the day? I think part of the reason is that we simply don't understand how important water really is.

From a weight-loss perspective, feeling hungry is one of the first signs of needing more fluids, which is why I would recommend drinking a large glass of water at the first sensation of hunger and then waiting twenty minutes to see if in fact you are still hungry. Simply put, I recommend drinking a full glass of water prior to eating because it will help to fill you up and you will eat less. Additionally, drinking a large glass of water first thing in the morning sets your day up for hydrating your body.

Water helps your blood cells carry oxygen and nutrients to your organs and also helps to carry the waste away. Water hydrates your body's cells and cellular functions. Your body needs and craves water all day—and that means every day. If you drink any beverage that contains caffeine, such as coffee, tea, energy drinks, sodas (including diet), or any type of alcohol, you will need to drink even more water. A perfect storm for dehydration is alcoholic drinks at night and coffee first thing in the morning. Let's face it, who hasn't done that at some point in his or her life?

If your body has lost 1–2 percent of its entire water content, you will feel hungry and thirsty, a sure sign that you need to replenish the lost liquids and you are on your way to dehydration. This prevents your body from performing its normal physiological functions. Mild dehydration can easily be treated, but if it reaches extreme levels, it can be life threatening and will require immediate medical attention.

The biggest problem, though, is the chronic dehydration that occurs over time and that has negative effects on your internal organs. This leads to kidney stones, cholesterol problems, constipation, poor liver function, joint pain, and muscle damage. Here is a link for thirteen symptoms of dehydration: http://bit.ly/2EE4M2DChronicDehydration

What Causes Dehydration?

It has been estimated that up to 75 percent of Americans are chronically in a state of dehydration. The biggest and most common cause of dehydration is that we are simply not drinking enough water: http://bit.ly/1RDkAxkDehydration Let's face it, we are busy people today. The more water we drink, the more we will need to use the bathroom, right? That takes time, and it may not be convenient.

Of course, there are many reasons for dehydration. Such as intense physical activity, commonly referred to as exercise. In the previous chapter I called it mobility, but you and I both know it is exercise. Many medications will also act as diuretics and may affect the crucial balance of sodium and potassium in our bodies, leading to dehydration.

Other causes include:

- **Diarrhea:** It prevents your intestinal tract from absorbing water from the foods and liquids that you consume.
- **Vomiting:** Common causes include foodborne illnesses, nausea, and alcohol poisoning.
- **Sweating:** Vigorous sweating may happen due to various reasons like fever and engaging in intense physical activity. Profuse sweating can also occur when you are working in hot conditions.
- **Diabetes:** Aside from having high blood sugar levels, some medications for diabetes frequently lead to excessive urination.
- **Frequent urination:** This can be caused by caffeine, alcohol, and certain drugs like antihistamines, blood-pressure medications, and antipsychotics.

Who Is at Risk of Dehydration?

Everyone and anyone can be at risk. Two groups of people who are especially prone to dehydration are mountain climbers and hikers. It is especially hard for them to stay hydrated because the increased air pressure in high-altitude places make people sweat more and breathe harder.

Athletes, especially those who are involved in marathons, triathlons, and cycling races, are predisposed to dehydration. The longer and more intense the exercise, the more you lose water in your body and you should be constantly hydrating. Top athletes in almost every sport are prone to dehydration, and it can affect the athlete's performance. Where there is an increase in dehydration, there will be a decrease in performance.

Infants and children are especially prone to dehydration since their bodies are more vulnerable to water depletion. Additionally, their need for water is greater than adults' need. A ton of research has been done on this. Children need more water! Check out this link with great video too: http://bit.ly/2G6V7yASmartKids

Elderly people are also at risk for dehydration since the actual thirst mechanism weakens as a person grows older. According to the BBC News, research reveals that many seniors are not getting enough water and becoming chronically dehydrated. Furthermore, as we age, we will lose our sense of thirst, and we simply forget to drink enough water. Additionally, people with dementia were found to have a six-fold increased risk for dehydration.

People with kidney disease, diabetes, cystic fibrosis, and adrenal gland disorders are also more prone to dehydration. People who drink alcohol on a regular basis will certainly be susceptible to chronic dehydration.

Benefits of Increasing Your Water Intake

- Helps you to lose weight by decreasing appetite, preventing overeating
- Increased cellular nourishment to our bodies' cells
- Greater flexibility
- Feeling more energy
- Smoother, better-looking skin; decreasing acne, blemishes, and dark circles under your eyes
- Increased vitality, concentration, alertness, and short-term memory

- Decreased joint pain and decreased frequency of headaches
- Better sleep and decreased mood swings
- Improved digestion and more efficient waste removal
- Improved detoxification
- Proper body-temperature regulation
- Increases your metabolism, which burns more calories
- Better immune response, decreasing allergies and asthma
- Room temperature water is better for hydration and absorption
- Cold water is good for cooling your body when exercising, slows digestion

What a list of great benefits from just drinking water and staying hydrated. Seems pretty simple to me. Drink up!

How Much Water Should You Drink?

In researching this exact question, I found numerous opinions from many very credible sources. The old "eight by eight" rule, meaning, drink eight 8-ounce glasses of water apparently does not have any actual research to support it, yet is certainly is a good start. Apparently, one size does not fit all in the category of water intake. So, let's take a closer look at what actually does matter: your body weight, the climate that you are in, how much you sweat, how much you exercise, how sedentary you are, and how much alcohol and caffeinated drinks you consume. Now things are getting complicated, aren't they? I don't like complicated.

Here are some basics for you to keep it simple. **For every pound you weigh, drink between one-half and one ounce of water.** So, if you weigh two hundred pounds, that means between one hundred to two hundred ounces of water every day! Check out this link for more information: http://wb.md/1NXsbvV. Next, take a close look in the bowl to check your urine color. If it is clear or very light yellow and has little odor, you are essentially well hydrated and probably doing just fine. Keep it up. The darker and more pungent your urine is, the more dehydrated your body is. We can actually make it that simple!

Since dehydration can be a life-threatening condition, it is important that you replenish your body with water immediately after you've lost a lot. Always bring a bottle of water with you during exercise or any physical activity, especially when the temperature is hot. Water plays such an immense role in your bodily functions, making it **an essential core energy source** for your everyday life.

It is especially important to pay close attention to people who have a fever, who are vomiting, or who are experiencing diarrhea, so they don't become dehydrated. Even though they may not feel like drinking water, they should be given water to replace the liquids that they've lost to prevent dehydration. An emergency-room visit due to dehydration for the most part is very preventable.

Drinking Sports Drinks Will Not Keep You Hydrated

Sports drinks are one of the most highly commercialized beverages today, from TV advertisements to popular athlete endorsements. Mainstream media makes it look like drinking these will keep you healthy and well-hydrated. Beverage companies advertise that sports drinks and energy drinks will help replenish the electrolytes and boost the energy in your body during exercise or outdoor activities. But the truth is that the ingredients of your favorite sports drinks will not hydrate or benefit you but may be detrimental to your health.

A typical sports drink contains high-fructose corn syrup (HFCS) and artificial sweeteners. It has two-thirds of the sugar content of soda and is thirty times more erosive to your teeth than water. HFCS causes negative health impacts like preventing the natural production of your body's human growth hormone (HGH). And again, if there is any caffeine in it, it will make you more dehydrated. Water should always be your go-to drink for hydration.

What about Diet Soda and Fruit Juice?

In addition to the artificial and neurotoxic sweetener aspartame, diet sodas also contain a larger amount of caffeine, even more than regular soda. As we have previously discussed, caffeine is a diuretic and will help to dehydrate you. So, please, pass on the diet soda for hydrating your body.

Commercial fruit juices are another sweetened drink that you must avoid because they do not have any hydrating properties and are loaded with sugar. For example, Minute Maid's 15.2-ounce bottle of orange juice actually contains a whopping 45 grams of sugar versus a can of Coke with 39 grams. For your body to get rid of the excess sugar that you consume, it must do two things: first, it must dilute the amount of sugar in your bloodstream by pulling water from your body, and second, it needs to get rid of the excess sugar by urination. This combination results in dehydration.

In addition, most processed fruit juices are made with little resemblance to what an actual fresh fruit juice would be. Commercial fruit juices are pasteurized, and their oxygen is removed to preserve them for a long time, which make the juices less nutritious. An expiration date of thirty days or more on store-bought fruit juice is a sign that it is heavily processed, so I encourage you to stay away from this type of beverage altogether.

Natural Thirst Quenchers for Preventing Dehydration

If you want to drink something more flavorful than water, you can opt for raw, organic green juice made from fresh vegetables. However, I recommend refraining from drinking juice with too many actual fruits in it, as there can be an excessive amount of the natural sugar, fructose. Fructose must be digested by the liver and breaks down into triglycerides, fat, and uric acid. Go for a green juice recipe that combines one or two fruits and larger amounts of greens like spinach, celery, or kale. That way, you can minimize your sugar intake and still get all the nutrients from the fruits and vegetables in their purest form.

Coconut water will serve as a great replacement for commercially sold sports drinks. It provides optimal health benefits due to the anti-inflammatory amino acids and antioxidants. A word of caution: coconut water also contains sugar, so you should drink it in moderation as well. I suggest drinking it preferably after a cardio workout, when you need to replace minerals and fluids.

The Key to Avoiding Dehydration: Listen to Your Body

Remember, always listen to your body. Once you feel thirst and the urge to drink choose clean, pure, filtered water rather than artificially sweetened beverages, which have negative effects on your health. No one can determine if you are dehydrated better than you. If you feel that you are already thirsty or have been sweating profusely, you need to replenish your body with water as soon as possible. Do not wait for significant symptoms to show up before you take action, since this can be life threatening.

A few years back my father passed out and was rushed to the emergency room. When I spoke directly to his attending physician he informed me that he was simply, dehydrated. Please, please avoid this. Remember that a healthy person urinates seven to eight times each day, so, if you're not urinating frequently, it means that you're not drinking enough water.

There is research that shows that drinking water in the morning immediately upon waking can have amazing therapeutic effects on a multitude of health conditions ranging from pain to asthma to cancer. This "water therapy" philosophy originates from ancient Ayurvedic medicine. The sages of India termed this therapy *Usha Paana Chikitsa*, which, from the Sanskrit, roughly translates to "early morning water treatment." It has long been known that drinking water first thing in the morning on an empty stomach purifies the body's internal system. An important result of this treatment is that it cleanses the colon, which makes the body absorb nutrients from food more efficiently.

In the 1970s, Dr. Fereydoon Batmanghelidj rediscovered this ancient knowledge and found through his own research that water can naturally heal us from diseases like high blood pressure, arthritis, asthma, autoimmune disorders, diabetes, and migraines. His research on over three thousand patients suffering from numerous diseases showed that they were helped using the healing powers of water. He reported his findings in the *Journal of Clinical Gastroenterology* and the *New York Times* "Science Watch" in June 1983.

In 1982, Dr. Batmanghelidj came to America and began his research on the effects of chronic dehydration on the human body. According to Dr. Batmanghelidj, the body's natural thirst signals are often mistaken for signs and symptoms of other illnesses. He states, "Over our lifespan, we can gradually become chronically dehydrated. By reversing that, we may be able to avoid unnecessary and invasive procedures, medications and chronic diseases." To learn more about Dr. Batmanghelidj and his work, here is the link: http://www.watercure.com.

Using Water to Improve Your Health

Right after waking up in the morning, drink at least one eight-ounce glass of fluoride-free and filtered water. If you're drinking water from a faucet and you have municipal water, chances are fluoride has been added to your water. Keep reading and you will learn more about fluoride later. You should consider drinking and bathing in water that is filtered or treated with a reverse osmosis system. Here are three keys from Dr. Batmanghelidj:

1. Begin drinking first thing upon waking and on an empty stomach.
2. Don't eat or drink for forty-five minutes after drinking the water. After forty-five minutes, you are free to eat and drink as you please.
3. Drink a glass of water a half hour before meals. Drink again two hours after each meal.

Here are some interesting facts about the benefits of water to help motivate you to drink sixteen ounces of water first thing in the morning: http://bit.ly/29FmvUpWaterHealth

1. It jump-starts your metabolism.
Drinking at least one large glass of water first thing in the morning has been shown to rev up your metabolism by a whopping 24 percent for the next ninety minutes.

2. You're dehydrated when you wake up.
After seven hours of sleep, chances are, you will wake up dehydrated. Drinking water helps make new muscle and blood cells and can increase the flow of oxygen, all of which are energizing.

3. Water helps your body flush out toxins.
"Your kidneys do an amazing job of cleansing and ridding your body of toxins as long as your intake of fluids is adequate," according to Dr. Kenneth Ellner, an Atlanta-based dermatologist. "Getting fluids into your body right after you wake up will help your body flush out toxins first thing in the morning." Flushing out toxins and impurities is even easier when you add fresh lemon to your glass. Lemon can increase the rate of urination, allowing for maximum enzyme function and helping to detoxify the liver.

4. Your brain tissue is 75 percent water.
When you are not properly hydrated, your brain operates on less energy, you feel drained, and you experience fatigue and mood fluctuations.

5. You'll eat less.
Studies show that people who drink a glass of water before every meal will lose weight, directly due to the feeling of being full.

6. It boosts immunity.
As cold and flu season is always just around the corner, it's vital to up your intake of water. If you tend to get sick often, you might not be drinking enough water. Staying hydrated can maintain the health of your lymphatic system, which directly affects how your body fights off infections. Studies have also shown that dehydration can cause increased cortisol levels, stress, and sickness.

Fluoride

I don't care what your dentist tells you, fluoride is highly toxic and is poisonous. There is enough fluoride in a tube of toothpaste to potentially kill a small child; that's because it is toxic and it's classified as a neurotoxin! Take a moment and read the label on your toothpaste. It says, "If accidently swallowed, get medical help or contact Poison Control Center right away." Fluoride is more toxic than lead. Do a thorough Google search for yourself or follow my links in this chapter!

Worse yet, we have toothpaste sitting out for our children to use without really knowing and understanding the facts about this toxic ingredient. Here is the link to the article published from the medical journal *Lancet* by Dr. Philippe Grandjean of the Harvard School of Public Health: http://bit.ly/22BEHnmFlourideToxic

Here is a list of absolute facts about fluoride:

- Fluoride was used in Nazi Germany by Hitler in the concentration camps to keep prisoners docile.

- Fluoride is a key ingredient in pesticides, specifically roach and rat poison.
- Fluoride is key ingredient in nerve gas.
- Fluoride is a toxic waste product from the production of aluminum and phosphates.
- Fluoride is a toxic waste product from the production of fertilizers.
- Fluoride is used in Prozac and Paxil.

This article, "Fluoride: The Most Toxic Substance for Humans," is full of references. I highly recommend reading it as it gives you the history of fluoride and the toxic effects: http://bit.ly/1srlrwoFluorideMostToxicSubstance Fluorine compounds or fluorides are listed by the US Agency for Toxic Substances and Disease Registry (ATSDR) as among the top 20 of 275 substances posing the most significant threat to human health.

Regardless of whether it helps to prevent cavities or not, you need to stay focused on where fluoride actually comes from, if it is healthy for our bodies, and most importantly, what in the hell is it doing in my tap water?

I always recommend doing your own research on topics of importance; that way you can make an actual informed decision on topics that are important to you. For me, health is one of my main priorities in life. When doing research on fluoride it becomes pretty easy to find the truth without much difficulty. There is some, shall we say, government cover-up in my opinion. The fact that fluoride, a toxic chemical, is being added into two-thirds of Americans' drinking water is a scam and a fraud and literally makes my blood boil!

Fluoride is a toxic waste by-product of the manufacturing of many products that we use and consume every day. The worst culprit—and the primary contributor to the fluoride dumped into our tap water—is from the fertilizer industry. Fertilizer is made by "strip-mining" or also commonly called "phosphate mining." These phosphates are used for fertilizer and are also turned into phosphoric acid, which is used in carbonated sodas such as Coke and Pepsi. Have you ever tried putting a penny into a glass of cola and watched to see what happens? Try it; you will be amazed how toxic it is. Coke is also a well-known rust remover. So why in heaven's name would you put that into your body?

Somehow, we Americans have been completely duped in to believing it is a great idea to dump fluoride into our drinking water. I find it very interesting that not all countries are proponents of adding fluoride to their water. Here is a partial list of countries that do *not* use fluoride in their drinking water: Austria, Belgium, China, Denmark, Finland, France, Germany, Greece, Hungary, Hong Kong, Iceland, Italy, Japan, Luxembourg, the Netherlands, Northern Ireland, Norway, Scotland, Sweden, and Switzerland. **The fact is, 98 percent of western Europe does not use fluoride in their water! Pretty interesting, isn't it?**

Here are the top reasons to avoid fluoride:

- Fluoride is a neurotoxin: http://bit.ly/1tnQYQBHarvardResearchChildren
- Fluoride causes arthritis: http://bit.ly/1VRH4lkCausesArthritis
- Fluoride increases bone fractures: http://bit.ly/22ZCgLCIncreaseBoneFractures
- Fluoride destroys sixty-two enzymes: http://bit.ly/1Ub9BzDestroysEnzymes
- Fluoride is toxic to the thyroid gland: http://wb.md/1Um84s4
- Fluoride calcifies brains' pineal gland: http://bit.ly/1YiJ7PYCalcifiesPinealGland
- Fluoride causes early female puberty: http://bit.ly/25SYZe8EarlyFemalePuberty
- Fluoride lowers testosterone in adult males: http://1.usa.gov/25PZt84
- Fluoride damages the kidneys: http://bit.ly/1UIBoorKidneyDamage
- Fluoride decreases our IQ: http://huff.to/1O7d578
- Fluoride increases ADHD: http://bit.ly/1TVPUPAIncreasesADHD

The documentary called *Fluoride: Poison on Tap* will completely blow you away! You will probably never want to drink tap water again unless you are lucky enough to live in a city that does not add fluoride. I highly recommend watching this; you will not be disappointed. Here is the link: http://www.fluoridepoisonontap.com.

Of the fifty largest cities in America. only six do not have added fluoride to their water: http://bit.ly/24lQYvISayNoToFluoride. Here is a detailed list of smaller cities that have rejected fluoridation since 1990: http://bit.ly/1r4MIUeRejectFluoride

Please, follow these links and watch the documentary. I believe you will come to the same conclusion as I have. I personally don't want any part of fluoride or added toxins and poisons to my water. I can't recommend enough to add a filtration system to your drinking water, and if you can, your house water as well.

Remember, if you don't use a filter for your water, then you become the filter. My research for high-quality water filtration that I personally use in my home can be viewed here: www.koehlerwellness.com/smart-water/.

The final chapter is coming up: "Your Support Team." Without having support in your journey to improving your health, it will be ten times more difficult. Following the guidelines in the prior chapters and committing to a clean-eating and mobility program takes a lot of commitment, dedication, and it really helps to know your why. Why do you want to do this? How will it benefit you? How will it benefit your family? Will it be easy? No, but I can guarantee you it will be worth it. Now, go find and build your support team!

Your Support Team

Support is defined in the Merriam-Webster.com dictionary as: "To promote the interests or cause, to give help or assistance to someone or something."

As social creatures by nature, and as group dynamics are, we can oftentimes do some fascinating and extraordinary things with support. I doubt I would have participated in the mid-1970s craze of streaking if my friends hadn't thought it was a good idea. When we are answering to other people, we can do things we can't typically do on our own, and it helps us rise to new heights!

That's the theory behind support or accountability groups. Groups unite around everyone achieving common goals. From my office, we have a private Facebook support group called **"Smart Health Experience."** This is an online group that is specifically for patients and clients who are on their health and weight-loss journeys. People will participate in one or more of our programs to achieve their goals. This group was designed for active participation, where we can post our latest victories, talk about how our workouts are doing, share our personal struggles, ask nutritional questions, and exchange ideas. For the most part we are all in there to support, inspire, and motivate one another. Frequently, there are personal struggles involved behind the scenes where one person has reached out to help another. The group has created friendships throughout the United States. Smart Health Experience is a private Facebook group—membership is by invite only—and has been going strong for over two years and has helped countless people along their journeys of becoming, "Health Warriors!"

Here are six steps to making your own accountability and support group succeed.

1. Pick a discrete and measurable goal.

You need an objective definition of success. "Be healthier" can't be tracked, but "eat five servings of fruits and vegetables per day" can. Big goals should be broken into discrete, measurable chunks. "Finish my dissertation," becomes, "work for an hour on my dissertation, three mornings per week." Any goal must be realistic. Life will always get in the way from time to time, and it can prevent people in your group from exercising every day. But hold yourself accountable to getting your workout in four times per week, and you will help to inspire yourself and others with motivation and momentum toward your health and weight-loss goals.

2. Pick people who truly want to lose weight and get healthier.

It's a funny thing about self-improvement: you would think it would be for people whose lives are a mess and need serious improvement. However, as I've learned, even people who have their lives "really together," still want to improve, learn new things, and take their lives and their health to the next level. Ultimately, you desire people in your group who will participate, who value discipline, and who enjoy helping others. Understand, though, as with all groups, there are highs and lows—people get busy, they fall off the wagon, and frequently, they will need a helping hand in getting back up.

3. Pick a leader, mentor, or coach.

Someone needs to "rally the troops" and occasionally call some people out when they haven't been active in the group. I personally was called out not too long ago. I must admit, I was a bit uncomfortable as I was the originator of the group. But truth be told, it was perfect timing, and it helped me back on track.

4. Aim for frequent communication.

Groups work best when people feel most connected. We, as a culture, walk around with the wrong mental picture in our minds about how people achieve. We don't succeed because we fear failure. Instead, the closer the group feels, the more likely it is that the individuals will achieve. We can and will do amazing things when we feel others are invested in our own accomplishments.

Consequently, groups where everyone simply checks in once a week with "success" or "fail" aren't going to be as motivational as ones where you're posting photos of you at the gym or eating your vegan lunch. You want to be able to share your struggles too. So set up an e-mail list or a private social networking group to facilitate this, and if you're a leader, post often. Hopefully others will too.

5. Allow for temporary failure.

Once you understand point four, you can understand this paradox of accountability and support groups. You need a way to make it OK for people to fail. Failure is not fatal. New habits are hard, and they take some time to develop, especially in our already busy lives. Since sharing struggles brings people together, you want a group where everyone brainstorms on how to help and solve problems with others. I have witnessed some mini-miracles in ours. When everything is going well for you and you are completely on track, you don't feel lonely; your own approval is enough. It's when things fall apart that you need the group to get you back on your feet. That is when the group can be the most beneficial for people.

6. Never reward laziness.

Someone who hits the gym three times one week when the group is pledging four times is in a different category from someone who doesn't go at all. Eventually, your group needs consequences if people aren't trying, because these free riders can upset group dynamics.

Use Peer Pressure to Your Advantage

There are ways to maintain your commitment to your goals, to keep your energy and enthusiasm high, and to feel like you are not in this alone. But to do this you must stay plugged in and connected with your group and participate. We're taught to think of succumbing to peer pressure as a flaw, but our dislike of letting others down can be a very powerful motivator.

A support group in which a small group of people share their goals, report back on their progress, and hold one another accountable is a fantastic way of getting things done and helping you reach your goals. You can create and set up your own support group. The bottom line is to help as many people as possible to achieve their goals.

To get serious results, you need to keep a few things in mind:

1. Don't (just) invite people you like.

It can be tempting to invite only your closest friends or those you get along best with; however, sometimes friends have a hard time offering and receiving constructive criticism. Objectivity from group members can be helpful when encouraging one another or calling one another out on lack of progress. Keep in mind that support groups may not suit everyone. Use social media and any interest groups you belong to and set clear expectations from the start. You are really looking for people who are serious about their journey.

2. Ensure everyone knows what to expect and what's expected.

When you invite people to join your accountability group, describe its purpose clearly so everyone understands the "psychological contract" of the group. Keep its focus front and center and be sure you are inviting people who will actively participate and stay committed to their journey.

A written description or group contract can also be helpful. For example, in our group we have used this phrase as a description, **"Will it be easy? Nope. Worth it? Absolutely."** Our group's goal is to encourage members to take action toward their goals and help to inspire and motivate others to do the same.

3. Take charge and keep everyone onboard.

Although the collective energy is what makes accountability and support groups work, someone does need to run the group. Someone must do the following:

- Structure the group the way you want it (this can always change).
- Ask the group for updates on how they are doing.
- Give a gentle nudge if a member hasn't checked in for a week or two.
- Ask members diplomatically whether they really want to be there if they've stopped checking in.

This requires drive, commitment, and probably a small dose of bossiness balanced with tact. It isn't for everyone, but there are advantages. For me, running my own group has meant that I'm not only committed to my goals as a member and as a leader, but I also know I'd be letting people down if I didn't put up the posts and encourage everyone to share their updates.

4. Keep your setup simple.

For example, put up a thread on Mondays saying something like "Accountability goals this week: Post your goals here!"

State the date so that people know which thread is the right one for the week and use a photo or a video to make it pop in their newsfeeds. On Sunday, you can post another photo with this: "Goals update: How did you do this week? Share with the group here!"

Sharing should make up 80 percent of the activity in the group. We try to keep it clean and distraction-free (no cat posts) so that our purpose—achieving our goals—is always at the heart of the group.

We've had the occasional thread on what kinds of workouts or meal plans have and haven't worked for people in the group, goal setting, and sometimes even odd questions. There will always be an opportunity to connect with others and to know you have a supportive community around you so you that you don't get derailed and come completely off the tracks with your goals.

5. Keep goals smart.

Help the group shape personal goals that are SMART:

Specific: Rather than "work out today," say "work out four days this week and go for three walks after work this week."

Measurable: Can you tell when you have achieved the goal? For example, completing a twenty-one-day quick weight-loss program or a sixty-day commitment program.

Attainable: The goal should always be achievable and attainable.

Relevant: Each small goal should relate to whatever your bigger goals are.

Time-bound: Be clear when you will complete each goal.

6. Agree on Consequences

The group's energy is crucial, so if you have people who have stopped checking in, ask them if they're still interested in being there. Try setting up the consequences of nonparticipation up front. For example, you can post a "rule" (pinned to the top of the Facebook page) that "if you don't post anything for two weeks (unless you've told us all you are on vacation or injured), then you can be gently released from our group."

Always be flexible with people. Everyone will have bad weeks where they don't achieve their goals, busy weeks where they fail to check in, a family crisis—we all know the drill. A small nudge may be just enough to help them refocus. If not, give them some private feedback to ask if they really want to be there. Communication is always the key.

Get Serious Results and Always Keep Your Sense of Humor

When run well, a support group can be fantastic for making progress over time on your own goals. It will force you to look strategically at the week ahead and establish your own priorities if you start to procrastinate. When and if you have a bad week—or even a bad month—you'll have a community of people who will support you and remind you that it's OK to wipe the slate clean. That way you can start each week afresh with a smile and an optimistic attitude.

Choose your group members wisely and set it up well, and you will be ready to achieve some serious results.

Do You Feel Like Your Health is Worth It?

Most experts agree that it's never too late to start getting healthier. True, you may have already done irreparable damage to your body. However, healthy living is the most powerful medicine of all. And, best of all, it doesn't require a prescription, and you won't have to concern yourself with adverse side effects—only the good ones. I realize that as we get older life sometimes can feel like an uphill battle, but I can assure you that with the right systems in place and the right support team, it can be done, and you can have fun doing it too.

Taking care of your own health is truly an inside job. You will need make daily decisions. You must put the work in, and you will have to remind yourself of why you wanted to do this and why it is important to you. We can provide you with all the systems and support, but the reality is, **it is up to you!** It will certainly take time, it will certainly take money, and it will certainly take work. You will learn more about yourself than you ever thought you would. You will more than likely stumble a few times before reaching your goals. I can tell you from experience, though, **it is so worth it!**

I'm going to tell the truth. You will probably be alive five years from now. You will probably be alive ten years from now. You may even be alive fifteen, twenty, and even twenty-five years from now. My question to you is: What do you want your life and your health to look like? Do you want to be tired all the time, with no energy, poor eating habits, and poor sleeping habits? Do you really want to wear that sleep apnea machine every night? When you were younger, did you really think that you would be this out of shape? Do you really want to be on all this medication? I don't think so.

I can guarantee you one thing: if you don't make the changes in your life and your lifestyle and you don't have your reason why firmly in place, your health will surely get worse as you get older. It's sad to say, but it's true. If we don't work on our health, it typically gets worse as we age. You must take an active role, learn the basics, get involved, and stay consistent. I realize this isn't for everyone. I get that.

There are plenty of people in this world who simply do not care about their health or their family's health. They are stubborn, lazy, think they know it all, and refuse to listen. There is no helping those people. We all know people like that. You are not one of those people; otherwise you wouldn't be reading this right now. I grew up a sick kid, I studied for seven years in college, and I've been in private practice for almost thirty years. I can say that without a doubt I am very healthy for a man in his fifties, and I'm on no medications.

I believe in my heart this path was chosen for me. Had I actually chosen to be that rock-and-roll star, bad-boy biker, engineer, or architect that I once wanted to be, I'm sure that I would still be sick today. More than likely, I would be overweight, taking the same medications (and probably more) and wondering why those shots don't seem to work anymore. I know what it's like to be sick, and I know what it's like to be healthy. I know that without putting in the work, your health will not get any better. It surely will decline and get worse as you age.

Again, it's up to you. You can join me in creating a healthier you, or what I call a "health warrior." Creating a healthier you will create a healthier family, creating a healthier community, and eventually, a healthier world. **I recommend starting *today* because your life may actually depend upon it.** If you want to schedule a consultation, please contact our office. I look forward to it!

Acknowledgments

I have had many mentors over the years who have inspired and motivated me to be the best me I can be. For this book, I want to acknowledge the following people for simply being their best and for assisting me when I needed them: Auntie Gail, Bo, Brandon, Brian, Bruce and Doreen, BarbaraSue, Dr. Christyne, David, Debbie, Emily, Dr. Fred, Dr. Rita, Hawk, Jim, Karen, Kim, Kristen, Kylie, Janet, Lindsay, Lolly, Lori, Mary, Matt, Mike, Pete, Dr. Randy, Dr. RoseMary, Sean, Sherry, Stacy, and Tyson.

About the Author

Dr. Craig Koehler grew up in the Central Valley of California in the city of Fresno. He has been in private practice in Huntington Beach, California, since 1992. As a young boy, he struggled with his own health problems, developing chronic allergies by age thirteen. This led to the overuse of prescription antihistamines, antibiotics, allergy shots, and finally, surgery. These medical procedures never solved or cured his condition, and he grew up as the sickly kid in school who was always sneezing, coughing, blowing his nose, and struggling to fit in. By the age of seventeen, he came to the realization that health did not come from a bottle of pills, from shots, and especially not from unnecessary surgery. His journey to find his own health resulted in him becoming a Doctor of Chiropractic at the age of twenty-six.

His personal mission, helping others with their health, has been paramount in his life. Through his own personal health research and working with his patients, he has come to a place where he feels he needs to share more of his knowledge. He feels that he must continue to educate not only his own patients, but also his community and anybody who is struggling with his or her own health, who needs the help and guidance that only an experienced professional can provide.

Dr. Koehler has found that many times people have developed so many poor health habits that they simply don't know where to start when it comes to turning their health around. Let's face it, we all know by now that our medical system is not making anybody healthy, especially when the traditional answer is the prescription of more and more medications.

Dr. Koehler has personally experienced some of his own family members dying of chronic diseases and has even seen fatal medical mistakes that always resulted in the devastation of the surviving family members.

There are reasons why our population in the United States is so sick. There is a reason why we are listed at number thirty-three of the healthiest countries in the world. This book will begin your journey to becoming more educated and can teach you the fundamentals of taking better care of yourself and making better, and smarter decisions for you and your family.

The next ten years are coming. How do you want your health to look? If you fall prey to the established medical system, it is typical and expected that your health will decline over the next ten years. It is Dr. Koehler's wish that your health will grow stronger over the next ten years. You know it will take some work on your part, as the "magic pill" theory has been proven ineffective. Together we can do this. Join us in this journey, but only if you truly want your health to improve.

Made in the USA
Columbia, SC
08 December 2019